LUCK OF
THE BEAN

• • • • • • • • •

A MEMOIR

BEN DOBSON

First Published in Great Britain in 2023

Copyright © 2023 Ben Dobson

ISBN 979-8-3902496-4-2 (paperback)

Cover Design by Creative Covers

Typesetting by Book Polishers

INTRODUCTION

FIRSTLY, THANK YOU for reading this far.

I would like to state that I am no more or less misfortunate than the next person. My story is no greater or lesser than anyone else's, it is just my story, and I'm grateful to have been afforded the opportunity to write mine.

I still don't have a grossly inaccurate Wikipedia page, nor do I grab headlines like Elon Musk or Kerry Katona, and I don't have an Instagram or Snapchat account or know whether I still exist on Facebook. I'm just a simple, ordinary man struggling to find peace and purpose who neither wants to be on 'Love Island' nor cares who wins this year 'Strictly Come Dancing'. If I were to relate to anyone on television, it would most probably be Mr. Bean. Coincidental, maybe, but my family nickname since birth has been 'Bean,' and it seems I am reluctantly destined to mirror my TV's namesake.

Finally, this book's intention is to celebrate life and its oddities. It's offered as a contribution, a connection, and a comfort. I hope it raises a chuckle or two and if you feel lost and rudderless, rest assured you're not alone.

ARE YOU SITTING COMFORTABLY?

'The world only goes round with misunderstanding.'
– Charles Baudelaire

FOR A NONDESCRIPT, dreary Tuesday afternoon, watching the butcher's apprentice being freed from beneath a frozen pig and driven away in an ambulance was worth the inevitable reprimand of returning late to a job I had loathed for five years. Stretched skeleton staff were still being worked into the ground as the workload, and head office expectations soared. The monthly internal newsletters attributed sales figures to 'happy coincidence,' repeating and urging employees to work harder and sell faster. Their message, minimum wage, and crippling hours implied that being a bookseller was a privilege and that our love for the written word and the company was our only reason for being. The disconnect between head office and the shop floor was huge and growing.

Once a year, our esteemed colleagues at head office would be reluctantly herded out to spend the day on the shop floor with the great unwashed in a pseudo gesture to bridge the yawning gap between 'them' and 'us'. For two consecutive years, they had spent their morning hiding in the stockroom, leaving at lunchtime without so much as a hello or goodbye. The follow-up newsletters advising us on how to up-sell and communicate effectively with punters became counter-productive. If anything, it only contributed to demoralising and angering an already demoralised, angered workforce.

I had lost all faith and passion for the role and entertained myself by writing provocative A4 notes for the attractive girl who worked in the jeweller's opposite, placing them amongst the children's books in the window. It always surprised me that regardless of what I wrote or how wholly inappropriate, we never received any comments or complaints

At the end of each day, it had become routine to stop at 'The Star' pub on the way to the train station with the usual determination to have just the one pint; just one to take the edge off another shitty day and always stumbled out into the night after they'd called time. The pub served two roles; a place to unwind but equally importantly, an escape from going home. It wasn't that home life was bad, it was just difficult living with my older sister and Mum. Three's a crowd and all that, and the prospect of spending every evening locked away in my room would only contribute in degrading my fragile mental health. Unable to enter into the local rental market on my income, even if I gave up the booze completely, I found refuge amongst other likeminded single men, all preferring company to the stinging silence of solitude.

My inebriated inability to understand the concept of time would often leave me staring blankly at the timetable board as I built up the willpower and strength for the 2-hour trek home, having missed the last train, again. The morning alarm would abruptly wake me to a nasty hungover and a medicated deep fatigue that lasted most of the day, abating in time for me to return to the pub that evening and start the whole cycle again.

My repetitive self-destruction strategy in protecting my mental health was of course, deeply flawed and inevitably led to damaging it anyway, which resulted in days at time being unable to leave my room, ironically putting me in the one place I had been trying to desperately avoid all along. On the days I couldn't face the world and certainly not converse with the public, it was company policy that staff must phone the store manager and explain their absence. Failure to do so would result in disciplinary action.

Confiding my deeply personal suicidal thoughts with a grossly unqualified peer over the phone seemed unfair to both parties.

With lengthy waiting lists and limited availability, access to mental health services wasn't expected, so when an NHS letter offering a workshop on 'Managing life' at Farnham Road hospital in Guildford dropped through the letter box, I eagerly accepted.

The day arrived, and after checking in, I followed the instructions to the room. I was the first to arrive, so opted to sit at the end of five chairs arranged in a semi-circle facing another chair. As others dribbled in, it was clear that some were in greater need of help than myself. One energetic, middle-aged hippy, wearing a fluorescent orange tie-dye tee-shirt and tatty jeans with hand-drawn flowers painted on, danced around to music which only she heard in her head. Another, in her 40's or 50's, sat beside me and wept inconsolably into a well-worn tissue. The other chap of similar age to me gazed around the room neurotically, as if expecting an unseen assailant to leap at him from the shadows at any moment. The final and fifth member of the group had wandered in looking lost, physically rather than mentally. When the door was closed immediately behind her, she meekly took the last remaining seat next to 'disco Sue', too embarrassed to leave.

No sooner had the doors been shut; they were flung open with such force the poor chap with the nervous disposition nearly crapped himself. In waltzed a diminutive buxom lady of African descent, wearing a floral dress so bright it made the fluorescent orange tie-dye tee-shirt look like it belonged in Victorian monochrome. As she made her way around us towards the solitary chair, her impossibly high heels resonated loudly through the wooden floorboards, drowning out the ambient background murmur. A red hat, about the size of a saucer, bobbed unpredictably on the crown of her head. She looked like she had come straight from or was going straight to the races; either way, her attire put the rest of us to shame. She stood facing us, opened her arms, and with an enormous, red-lipsticked grin and the strongest Caribbean accent I've ever heard, addressed us:

'Well, hello, my lovelies. How are we today? Welcome to Marion's workshop on "Managing life." I'm Marion. We're in a safe space.'

She was lovely. Even from her laconic introduction, she radiated warmth, kindness, care, and compassion. She was an earth mother and one of those rare people who, when they wrap you in a duvet of a hug and tell you everything will be okay, you believe them.

We then, as a group, explored the word 'emotion' or, more accurately, due to her audience's indifferent participation, she described emotion and then gave examples. When she mentioned grief, the weeping lady fumbled and fought through her pockets to retrieve another equally sodden, limp tissue.

The next topic in Marion's workshop was meditation. Not any meditation, but a guided one, and one that I'll remember for the rest of my life. (This dialogue was noted in the car park immediately following the workshop and was as accurate as I could remember.)

'Meditation can help with difficult emotions. When we get angry, anger is an emotion, meditation can help calm us down. I want to take you on a meditation, my lovelies. Close your eyes and come with me to a happy place, I want you to inhale…and let it all out…good…good, feel the air rush in…and out…that's it… in…out…in…out…now I want you to imagine yourself in a beautiful place…a safe place…a golden, happy place, a place of piss…'

I was straight back in the room, eyes wide open, thinking I must have misheard her.

'Good…good…that's it…feel the piss…feel it flow over you…warm…golden piss…in…out…'

Despite her purest intentions, unfortunately, her accent had given the meditation and workshop a whole new meaning. As I sat there, trying to hold my laugh in like a 6-year-old girl, she continued…

'Let the piss flow over you…through you…warm…golden

piss…can you feel the piss…I can feel piss…are you feeling my piss…good…I feel piss all over me…'

I glanced at my peers to see whether anybody else had noticed. The other chap had stopped scanning the room and was staring at her, mouth ajar in disbelief; the sobbing woman had buried her head in her hands and had begun gently rocking, 'disco Sue' seemed to be enjoying it, giggling and occasionally clapping, whilst the lost lady had mustered the courage to tip-toe her way towards the exit.

By the end of Marion's well-meaning workshop, I had learned very little about 'Managing life,' but in her own unique way, she had changed our lives; I doubt the five of us will ever be able to read or hear the word peace without thinking of her guided meditation, and to me, that can only be a good thing and makes me warm inside; my trouser leg.

Determined to find work away from high-street retail and break the vicious circle I'd found myself in, I began scouring the internet looking for all other career options. One website that popped up offered a voice-over workshop day in London where an industry producer would, for a small fee, give an honest opinion on the marketability of the voice. With nothing to lose and short of any other ideas, I booked a place.

The day was a mixed bag. I had a decent showreel, and the eagerly anticipated email confirmed that my voice, did indeed, had a certain marketability. However, I had yet to learn how technical and competitive the industry would be or the jaw-dropping expense of setting up a virtual home studio and the costs of training. Another sizeable obstacle was the intense competition. A host of A-listers and professionally trained voice-over actors audition for the bigger pay-outs with the successful candidate usually offered one of two payment methods; a one-off fee or a royalty every time the voice is used. One BMW campaign paid the voice of their commercials a six-figure sum for less than 20 seconds of dialogue. For optimum voice quality, unthinkable sacrifices like cheese and dairy products would have to be made, which, considering at least two of my three meals a day consist of cheese, deemed that career out of the question.

The following day, I returned to work and happened to be speaking to Debbie, a postmistress who worked in the adjoining post office, about the previous day. She laughed and told me about her blonde-haired, blue-eyed brother, who was still living well off Asian royalties, having starred in an international Bounty chocolate bar advertising campaign 20 years ago. I can vividly recollect that advert too. A muscular, man Friday character walked along a pristine, white-sanded beach on a paradise island with the sunsetting when in slow motion, a coconut falls and splits open, revealing a wrapped Bounty bar.

When we were reduced to one staff member on the shop floor who was responsible for till targets, phoning through customer orders, stocking the shelves, customer enquiries, merchandising of current campaigns, cashing up from the day before, gift wrapping (at Christmas), embargoed titles and research of upcoming titles I'd had enough. Heaven forbid the bookseller should ever need the toilet. They had taken enough piss out of me in my five years of service and this new stream-lining of skeleton, skeleton staff was the two fingers that broke my back, leading me to tender my month's resignation.

Without purpose or direction, I saw out my final days in much the same I had conducted most of the previous five years, by heading to the pub every evening. But, in a timely twist of fate, it seemed that the countless hours and the hundreds of pounds I'd invested in ruining my liver, hadn't gone unnoticed. During my various ramblings and forgotten introductions, I had met a couple who owned an events company and hearing of my upcoming unemployment, invited me to lunch the following day. The long-overdue final day ended with emotional drunken goodbyes to my colleagues and setting a massive new record for the slowest, least direct walk home.

THE ART OF SELLING WITHOUT SELLING

'In Germany, they all thought I was a bit mental, very emotional.' – **Jürgen Klopp**

THE LONG, LANGUID liquid lunch with the both of the directors in a gastro pub, and the most informal job interview I've ever attended, ended with me accepting the enviable position of Sales director of the U.K. Pool and Spa Exhibition at the N.E.C in Birmingham. The hours of slow, tipsy, midday intoxication was an early glimpse of what the position and future held.

Keeping the promise to myself that I wouldn't work in high street retail again, the events company's H.Q was located *just off* the high street. Due to council regulations, the premises had to be a retail outlet, so in a stroke of genius, my employers had partitioned the space into one enormous open-plan office and a tiny, 3m x 1m 'shop front', selling a very limited, random range of infused olive oils.

Four of us worked in the office, equipped with a small seating area and a kitchenette at the back, and as my desk was closest to the inter-connecting 'shop' and I had retail experience, I was the designated 'shop-keeper.' My categorically incorrect sales pitch that we only stocked 100% organic, 'free range' olive oil usually saw confused customers leave empty-handed. On the odd occasion that someone wanted to purchase a half-litre bottle, the office would descend into utter chaos as we weren't prepared take any means of payment. We didn't possess a card reader, so patrons were asked to pay cash, but we didn't have a float either, resulting in the customer replacing the bottle on the shelf to gather dust and wishing us a trite good day as they closed the door behind them, baffled.

We worked on our own individual expos, selling space and additional extras such as lanyards and program sponsorship to industry companies worldwide. My expo was held domestically, so I had few problems communicating with the venue and most of my clients. In contrast, one of my colleagues organising a technology exhibition in Delhi would have to work with different time zones, regularly travelling out to liaise with his Indian counterpart, and always returning with Delhi belly and the need to self-isolate for a week. He was a three-piece tweed-wearing 20-year-old going on 60 who had spent much of his childhood trotting around on one of his father's polo-horses or in the back of a chauffeur driven Bentley. India really had been quite the eye-opener on how the other 99.9% of the world's population lives.

As I was a newbie to the industry, the directors, Sam and Hannah, decided that it would be beneficial for me to travel to the beautiful, industrial town of Stuttgart to experience how the Germans organised an exhibition similar to my baby happening in a few months.

I had essentially been hired in an organisational and sales role, so when I eventually arrived at Heathrow, an hour late for my flight, having survived a 360° spin on a wet, early morning M25, the omens didn't bode well and hadn't done my underwear any favours either. Miraculously, due to adverse weather conditions, Lady Luck had delayed my flight by 2 hours, redeeming what would have been a catastrophic first professional impression.

Sam collected me at Stuttgart Airport, and with my trailing luggage tripping everyone in my wake, we made our way over the narrow causeway to the exhibition hall and the largest indoor space I'd ever been in. I'm not new to huge venues, I've done my fair share of long-distance viewing at live shows, but this place made the O2 look like Harry Potter's cupboard under the stairs.

With 20/20 vision, I could barely see the roof let alone the far wall. A clock displayed two different time zones, and an array of international flags the size of tennis courts fluttered overhead as far as the eye could see. Sponsored blimps were dotted throughout the ginormous hall, purposely designed and located for lost souls to regain their bearings.

We arrived at our modest 'UK Ambassadors' stand, which seemed to serve no other purpose than for luggage storage, parked my one-wheeled, meandering menace of a suitcase and set off doing the rounds with my freshly printed business cards in hand and an ambitious sales spring in my step.

An hour later, I had barely made it a third of the way around the building, not only due to the enormity of the place or the mother of all blisters which had totally engulfed my right heel but because of the stunning selection of complimentary alcoholic beverages on offer. Every stand seemed to have a fully stocked bar with an eager barman ready to recharge bottomless glasses, so instead of approaching it professionally and harvesting potential clients, I had one drink and was off, keeping my business cards safely tucked away in my pocket and my profession ambiguous.

The stands that did the swiftest business were those tended by attractive, scantily-clad women. A few of the more extensive stands even had an hourly show where five or six bikini-wearing women in heels would parade down a narrow catwalk, gyrate around a temporary, shiny pole, and exit stage in a cloud of dry-ice to various grunts of approval from the exclusively male audience. It was moths to a flame. Some men had listed show times in note books and arrived 15 minutes prior to the show started, taking the seats directly beside and slightly below the catwalk, guaranteeing themselves the seediest points of view as they shoved in foot-long bratwursts and shook their empty glasses at the busy barman. As soon as it was over, they would melt away only to return an hour later, with absolutely no intention of doing any business other than their lustful own.

When Sam found me in a small, remote dry sauna, sharing

a bottle of peach schnapps and a cigar with two splendid moustaches and their proud Austrian owners, I braced myself for an immediate firing and the next plane home. Instead, I was gently reminded of my professional objective before he calmly left, leaving me to drain the bottle, say my enthusiastic German goodbyes and head off on my merry way again, hunting for my next bottle of schnapps to enjoy with other hairy strangers in an absurdly tiny space.

At the end of the day, after the doors were closed to the public, some of the more prominent companies which had the sound systems and fully functioning, water-filled spas sent the dancing ladies home, then completely de-robed and sat fully naked in, on, and around the spas, often with a cigar in one hand and always with a drink in the other.

Even through one blurry eye, the sight of dozens of naked EU members did seem somewhat surreal, although that didn't prevent me from stripping down to my pants, folding my suit, climbing in, and joining them. It was difficult to ignore the distinct whiff of German sausage that hung heavy in the air.

I spent an hour drunk and lost, wandering around in my pants and socks, carrying my wounding shoes with my suit and shirt draped over my forearm. The cleaners looked thoroughly bewildered when I asked them for directions in my finest, drunken German. My phone's battery had died hours previously, so when Sam found me, I took it as a favourable sign Lady Luck was still looking after me.

With the exhibitor's formal meal taking place in an hour, I didn't have time to return to the hotel to change, so after a quick rummage through my suitcase for a clean shirt and a pair of pants at our obsolete stand, I was ready and raring to go.

Adjoining the great hall was a smaller one, where dozens of circular tables had been made-up of crisp, white linen and ladened with burnished cutlery for three courses. A 12-piece brass band wearing traditional lederhosen played traditional 'Oompa Oompa' hits on a raised stage. Next to the smaller hall was a reception room where delegates had gathered for pre-dinner drinks and, bizarrely, to play fairground games. All the classics were there; bucking bronco, pop the balloons with darts, hammer and bell, the claw game, and even a coconut shy. There was also enough free booze to keep the Irish happy for a month. Attractive Jägermeister reps circulated the room, directly delivering the loopy juice into waiting mouths, from a heavy-duty, pump-action modified water pistol, like a blackbird feeding it's young.

My competitive enthusiasm rubbed off on Sam, who really should have been more responsible and returned me to our table, but instead positively threw down the gauntlet and joined me in fierce competition against any willing German as a matter of national pride. We remained unbeaten on the hammer and bell game, commanding a crowd five or six deep every time someone challenged us; we successfully grabbed a whoopee cushion in a Perspex ball from the claw game, stayed on the bucking bronco for longest, and popped all the balloons in the dart game, earning us a five-foot, green inflatable alien. We were invincible. As for the coconut shy, well, being an active member of the mighty Witley cricket club, there was only ever going to be one winner. Also, I'd never seen a sozzled German throw a ball, but it was humiliatingly obvious they hadn't attended one of Mr. Hickman's monster Thursday afternoon fielding sessions. By the time my right shoulder had gone numb, we had more coconuts than the shy, so to ease the rising tensions, donated our winnings back to the shy, which earned us a triple pump from the Jager blunderbuss. Asking for three more pumps was my last memory of the night.

I IGNORED THREE internal calls and was rudely brought into the day by loud, constant knocking on the door. Still a little pissed, very hungover, thoroughly confused, and with a massive bruise on the right side of my ribcage, I refused what I thought was efficient housekeeping. The knocking got louder, and with it, my insistence that their services weren't required, and yet it carried on. I struggled to the door and opened it to an old, small angry man who with narrow eyes and a sharp tongue introduced himself as the director's father and the company's legendary founder. In no uncertain terms, he colourfully informed me that he had been waiting in the foyer for over an hour after getting up at 4 am to catch the 7 am flight. My profuse, slurred apologies fell on deaf ears, quite literally, as I later found out. He gave me 30 minutes to 'sort myself out' before he left in the waiting taxi. Mysteriously and disconcertingly, my suit and shirt were neatly folded on a chair I'd never seen, next to a bed I'd never seen, in a hotel room I'd never seen, in a hotel I didn't know the name of.

By 10 am, I was in the taxi sitting next to a silently seething old man, holding my ribs, barely able to see or stand, and castigating my own stupidity. Overnight, my original blister had now grown its own blister, but what troubled me most wasn't my battered body; it was the complete amnesia of the night before. The agonising, 20-minute ride staring out of the window jolted nothing, so when we arrived at the venue 2 hours late, he was no happier, and I was none the wiser.

The first worriment that things were amiss was the familiarity of some of the stand holders. The rub of my shoe's leather had induced a pronounced limp, and while I struggled to keep up with the purposeful pensioner, occasional holders offered up their hands for me to slap as I shuffled by. The more hands I slapped, the more my anxiety grew.

I arrived at our stand fearing the worst, but again, rather than ripping me a new one, the directors seemed pleased to see me, even wishing me a smiley good morning. My eye was caught by the 5-foot, partially inflated, green alien reclining on one of the chairs in the seating area, looking like I was feeling and jogging partial, uncomfortable memories. A black coffee was thrust into my hand before I was led to a seat and shown the first of four recordings on Sam's phone.

The footage was shaky but unmistakable. Blindfolded with my tie on the back of the bronco, initially with two hands, then one, then very briefly none before I was catapulted off so violently, I was thrown over the surrounding protective cushions straight onto the concrete floor. The clip ended with people gathering around my crumpled, lifeless body. The bruised ribs made perfect, painful sense now. I held my head in my hands. He then slanted his phone towards me and tapped play again.

Still blindfolded with my tie and shirt all but one unbuttoned, I was standing at the hammer and bell game in front of about 100 onlookers, absolutely pissing sweat. With the crowd giving a German countdown from 5, my first attempt missed completely. In truth, it wasn't close. Not only did I miss, but the rubber hammer came down at such an angle that it ricocheted off the floor into the shin of a plump, middle-aged woman who, considering the state I was in was standing far too close. Unperturbed by my first failure and unaware of the causality it had caused, I demanded another go while readjusting the tie back over my eyes. The crowd erupted as a pair of rogue, masculine hands entered the frame to manoeuvre my hips into position. The German countdown from 5 started again. My second attempt hit home, sounding the bell loud and clear to thundering applause. As I removed my tie to take an appreciative bow, I dropped the hammer, which bounced back into the same shin of the reeling woman I had injured on my first attempt. I was oblivious and obediently opened up to be rewarded with a double pump from the Jägermeister reps.

I started to feel unwell. I needed a cold coke.

In the third recording, I had progressed to wearing my tie around my head like Rambo, shirt fully unbuttoned and billowing behind me, hairy chest exposed, and nipples protruding proudly. I also had the alien clinging to my back, its skinny arms tied around my neck, its head bobbing on my right shoulder. I don't know why but I had taken it upon myself to run around the tables, high-fiving as many hands as possible with the alien's hand. It was clear by some sauerkraut faces not everyone was finding it as entertaining as I was.

The fourth and final recording was especially tough to watch. While most attendees were digging into their formal sit-down meal, I was completely shirtless, still wearing my tie around my head, still piggybacking the alien and leading a 40-strong line in a conga around the dining hall. I watched and wilted as we weaved through the tables, collecting willing strays on the way. When we made our way up the stairs onto the stage, there were far too many moving parts. Climbing stairs while doing the conga to the beat of a brass band, shitfaced, is not recommended. Despite having their stage invaded, the band played on; until one chap about ⅔ down the line, who was a dead ringer for the late Alan Rickman, got his timings all wrong, veering off into the drums and drummer, taking the tail with him. I was still blissfully unaware of the mayhem unfolding behind me, as I was having my own issues leading the front ⅓ down the stairs at the other end of the stage. The footage finished with me and my alien dancing my flock into the games room as band members fished Alan Rickman and a couple of others out of the demolished drum kit.

Sam told me he later found me slumped asleep against the claw game, shirtless, tie around my head, and still being loyally embraced by the alien. While Sam collected my discarded clothes and took me back to the hotel, Hannah was having a field day reaping valid contact details from some curious, some angry, but mostly concerned diners, therefore deeming the evening to be a tremendous success. Any PR, even the most crushing, is still worthy PR.

I spent the next 7 hours trying to keep water down and hobbling horribly due to the red raw hole where my heel used to be, dishing out high fives and apologies in equal, awkward measure, feeling like I might die at any moment. By the time I collected my wonky suitcase and been dropped off at the airport, I was a shadowy ghost of my former self. If I thought that was the end of my self-induced hellish nightmare, I was mistaken, for Lady Luck had one more trick up her abundant sleeve.

Having arrived at Heathrow an hour late for my outgoing

flight, and in shock after seeing my life flash before me on the M25, I hadn't been paying much attention to where I'd parked my car, and as my ticket was no longer in my suit jacket pocket, presumed lost in Stuttgart, I had few clues to go on. I took four airport shuttle buses to 3 car parks, revisiting one car park twice. I had removed my right shoe for blister relief, and the one wheel on my suitcase was no longer remaining. Four hours after touching down in Blighty, I was no closer to finding the whereabouts of my car and began weighing up which one of the bus shelters would be most comfortable for the night. Maybe it was the solitary tear rolling down my cheek, or more probably, it was the sight of a grown, suited man wearing one shoe, dragging a fraying suitcase that caught the attention of the passing security patrol. After listening to my story suspiciously, he agreed to help locate my car. An hour later, he was starting to lose patience, understandably. It was on the way back to the bus shelter, where I'd mentally prepared myself for a night on a row of plastic chairs, I saw her golden roof glisten in the intermittent moonlight. I was overwhelmed. The previous 48 hours had finally taken their toll, reducing me to an unbridled mess. When two long strands of snot dangled from my nose and became tangled in my fingers, the security guard had seen enough and reached over to open my door.

The final kick in the nuts was the animated argument I had with a seriously disinterested customer service advisor, who, after fining me for my lost ticket, helpfully advised me to 'go fuck myself'.

Stuttgart had taken a chunk out of me, quite literally, regarding my right heel, and to this day, I still gag at the sight of Jägermeister and the smell of German sausage, or is it the other way around? My loyal partner, the alien, also made the journey back and sat, slowly deflating in the office seating area, constantly reminding me of one of my most mortifying nights.

In comparison, my show at the NEC was like attending an Amish funeral.

-     No fairground stalls.
-     No brass band.
-     No formal dinner.
-     No Jägermeister sharp-shooters.
-     No hourly pole-dancing.
-     No naked sit-ins.
-     No lasting kidney damage.
-     No awkward high-fives the morning after.

The only commonality was my giant blisters.

The atmosphere was dire since I'd only sold half the space available. None of the bigger stands with their sound systems or pole-dancing ladies had booked, so all that could be heard was the occasional clatter of stands being erected and corrected and the reversing beeps of forklifts as they shuttled pallets around behind the scenes. There were several entirely vacant rows which were more likely to see tumbleweeds pass down them than members of the paying public. Footfall numbers were way below what I had quoted and the exhibitors were only too happy to remind me of it.

By the end of the second and final day, my clients confirmed that it had indeed been the worst Pool and Spa expo they'd ever experienced, both in trade and atmosphere. They also categorically told me they would not be attending any future events.

The following week I was back behind my desk with the phone to my ear, staring at the alien and struggling to sell space for the next year's doomed expo. I found it particularly difficult to hit my targets when I had no confirmed dates, no confirmed venue, and no costings. Something had to give, and that something was me handing in my resignation.

It had been a whirlwind of an education. I miss those guys, but I especially miss my wingman, dance partner, affectionate hugger and loyal friend. I just hope they remember to inflate him from time to time.

TAKE THAT

'Revenge is always sweet, it's the aftertaste that's bitter.'
– Joshua Caleb

STILL CLUELESS ABOUT what path to take, I went about registering with several Godalming employment agencies and was jubilant to hear their optimism about finding me my perfect vocation. Although I've spent nearly all my life trying to figure out what to do, I was eager to see which industry they thought my skills were bested to.

I went into the first interview I ticked all the boxes for most of the available positions advertised on their website, and they'd be begging me to name my terms for any of them. Perhaps not surprisingly, they didn't entirely concur. Instead, it turned out that I was over-qualified for all of my preferred choices, but not for envelope stuffing in a village shed on minimum wage. It seemed I was perfectly qualified to do all the tasks that a robot programmed by a five-year-old could manage. Rather than enduring 40 hours a week being paper-cut, the only other position I was suitable for was arranging leather jackets into size order in a warehouse on an obscure industrial estate outside Guildford.

After five days of fighting through a giant cow wardrobe, I wondered whether the bookshop had any vacancies. Two weeks in, and I'd had enough. Judging by the recruitment consultant's reaction, I had surpassed their expectations on how long I had stayed and then was briskly offered envelope-stuffing again.

The next role I accepted was based just on the outskirts of

Godalming, in a converted stable block, where a red-headed and rosy-cheeked man in his 60s and a woman in her 30s sat behind vast desks and Apple Macs at opposing ends, working in silence. It was so quiet that within two weeks, I could accurately distinguish between my boss's two waste requirements simply by the noises of his inner workings. It was a three-month, numbing telephone placement selling sponsorship for education tradeshows, accumulating contacts for future tradeshows, compiling attendance numbers, and answering the odd, rare inquiry from the public. The first month was fine. Ponderous but fine, and I had grasped enough that my boss was confident to leave me in the office while he travelled to do business at other, professionally-related tradeshows.

I hadn't had anything to do with the lady at the other end of the office until the second time my boss went away, when she left me a letter to email with a yellow post-it stuck on explaining she was short of time. As a one-off, I duly obliged and thought nothing of it. The third time my boss left, the door had barely shut when two letters and a hand-scribbled timetable with another yellow post-it note attached at the top that had the message 'Excel' appeared on my desk. Before I could question or clarify anything, she was gone, out the door and away. I still didn't even know her name.

I spent the next three days diligently watching Youtube tutorials on building spreadsheets, and as I wrestled with the very basics of computers, my telephone work fell behind, earning me a stern talking to on my boss's return. I don't know why I bit my tongue and kept quiet; I suppose I thought it a little churlish to blame her directly; besides, I was expecting her to come to my aid. But as he tore into me, I noticed her readjusting and hiding behind her screen, making herself as small as possible.

The next time my boss ventured out, he gave me clear instructions as to what was expected of me, and sure enough, no sooner had his car left the car park than another bundle of papers popped up on the corner of my desk. We hadn't yet had a conversation. In two weeks. With only three of us in the office. I swung around in my chair and, glaring at her, said,

'You are joking, aren't you?'

She carried on, completely ignoring me, and sat motionless behind her screen.

'What the fuck's going on?' I not so politely enquired.

Nothing. She absolutely refused to talk or even look at me. I tried to recall what I'd done to offend her, whether it was my shirt, shoes, or insistence on not wearing trousers on Thursdays; whatever it was, her silence and my apparent invisibility weren't helping matters.

'Hey? What's going on? I'm doing all this extra work,' I tried again, in a softer tone.

Movement. Just when I thought I'd broken through, she grabbed her coat and stormed out of the office, leaving me huffing and puffing, asking myself what the fuck was happening? If I thought phoning my boss and throwing blame was childish, what I did next was positively infantile, and I'll be the first to admit that. Something broke in me when I saw her turn out of the car park. I went into autopilot in the kitchenette, took the lid off the sugar holder, and mixed in flour which every kitchen in the country seems to have, and salt from a dozen takeaway paper packets I'd found forgotten at the back of one of the cupboards. I had fully expected to be walking out then and there, happily seeing neither again, but Lady Luck seized her opportunity to teach me otherwise.

Gathering my coat from the back of my chair, I heard not one but two cars drawing up and parking outside. My boss was the first to come busily through the door, closely followed by the woman with no name, clearly upset.

'Ben, I think there's been a misunderstanding somewhere along the way. Lucy has just texted me saying you've had a go at her. It sounds like the agency didn't fill you in, did they?'

'Err…no…I don't think they did'. A slow sense of foreboding seeped through me.

'Right, that explains it. I was quite clear in my instructions to them.' He perched himself on the corner of my desk and turned to the woman,

'Lucy dear, would you mind putting the kettle on, please, and we'll have a chat which the agency should have had with you'.

I sat rooted to my chair, watching in slow-motion horror as Lucy picked up the kettle and having felt its satisfactory weight, flicked it on.

'So, what they should have told you, and I can't believe they didn't, was that you're covering for Lucy, my daughter, as she recovers from complications following a tonsillectomy. She usually does what you're doing, but, well…long story short, she's on an extended course of antibiotics for a particularly nasty infection which makes it painful to talk and to swallow. It's been especially bad these last couple of weeks, hasn't it my dear?'

Lucy, with her back to us, said nothing and dropped three tea bags into three mugs.

'Plus, you're quite quiet anyway, aren't you?' He continued, gazing at her adoringly.

She stood silently and patiently waiting for the kettle to boil. I was also lost for words. My mind was too busy furiously racing for a realistic reason to suspend the tea-making process, and while he watched her pour the water into the mugs, I searched for anything that would disrupt proceedings. A ping of an email, a wrong number phone call, a bird flying into the window, the wish for a sudden bout of diarrhoea, but nothing came, even after pushing. As I watched her squeeze the tea-bags in the mugs before discarding them, I wondered how karma would surely repay me.

Just when I resigned to a well-deserved kicking, a criminal record, and a leper-like status around town, Lady Luck came to my rescue at the eleventh hour. We watched as she heaped two spoons of sugar/flour/salt into the mugs and added the milk.

'Oh no! It looks like the milk is on the turn. I only bought that yesterday.' He said disapprovingly. 'Unless you want yours without milk and just sugar?'

I couldn't believe it. Never have I been so grateful for the mysteries of chemistry I don't understand.

'No, I'm good, don't you worry; thank you anyway.'

'Are you sure? It's no trouble.'

'Definitely sure, thank you.'

Now that I had wriggled out of being hoisted by my own petard, my attention fell to Lucy's next move. There was a moment's hesitation as she sniffed the milk and dithered, thinking about a second attempt before she screwed the lid back on the milk, placed it on the counter, and poured away the contents of her mug.

I spent the rest of the afternoon with my arse nervously twitching whenever either of them went anywhere near the kitchenette and spent an hour after work driving to and from a garage for a replacement packet of sugar, thanking Madame fate for her timely intervention.

I saw out my contract without any further vengeful, regretful acts. As the weeks passed, Lucy's throat improved and returned, revealing her as a thoughtful, kind and considerate creature.

ACHTUNG BABY!

'I've been lucky to have survived balloon trips, boating trips, you know, a lot of rather foolish things in my life, so I was definitely born under a lucky star' – **Richard Branson**

ANY 5.30 AM alarm is a rude awakening. Even the ones that wake you for something nice. Having been aborted twice due to inclement weather conditions, it was third time lucky that a brief girlfriend and I got the go-ahead that we'd be reaching for the stars in a hot air balloon.

She had booked our aviation adventure months previously and was so excited that she insisted we turned up at the launch site with an hour to spare. As she stared into the early morning summer sky with a childlike wonderment on her face, I stood shivering, thinking that maybe I had come underdressed in my threadbare, Fruit of the Loom tee-shirt and linen trousers for the 2000ft, hour flight.

Our party consisted of a young, in love, hand-holding lesbian couple, an endearing old couple with binoculars around their necks, and a sixty-something-year-old man escorting his impossibly ancient mother around by the arm.

The middle-aged, moustached pilot went from one group to the next, cheerfully introducing himself. To each party, it was the same:

'Good morning, good morning, hello, I am your pilot today. My name is Herman from Düsseldorf, or as my English friends call me, Herman ze German'.

Unbeknownst to me, hidden away in the small print was, according to Herman, the agreement that passengers were expected, 'where physically possible, to assist the pilot in erecting the balloon.' As I looked around at my fellow flying companions, I realised I had a lot of work on my hands. And so, while I ran around like a headless chicken, wrestling with unravelling the red nylon, the rest of the passengers stood by, watching on behind their phones in sensible overcoats and bobble hats.

I was the last to scramble into the basket feeling as if I'd just had a full workout with my sweat-sodden tee shirt clinging to me. Luck would just so have it that I found myself in the very opposite corner to my girlfriend, nullifying any chance of any sweet romance or mile-high conquests. In the one doomed effort to get closer to her, I only succeeded in getting wedged between the barely alive old woman and Herman, directly beneath the balloon's brutal burner.

Standing 6'2 naked and 6'4 in the occasional Friday night Geisha geta, I spent most of the flight feeling like I was wearing the balloon as a giant punishment hat. The sole attempt at a toast with my girlfriend from afar only resulted in me spilling cheap prosecco on the old lady's head and wearing the rest down my front, refreezing my nipples to my damp tee shirt.

Eventually and thankfully, our Luftwaffe ace informed us that we were on our final descent and as the basket had shifted during flight, I found myself free from sniffing prosecco off the top of the old lady's permed hair and burning my head and, for the first time, some space to peer over the edge and marvel at the purple and yellow patchwork heathland stretching out beneath us.

At last, a long-awaited sense of peace.

I'm not sure who spotted the seven-foot, caged sapling and the only vertical sign of life first, but as soon it was made known, there was a dreadful inevitability with what was about to unfold. The irony of crashing into the only living tree for miles around was neither lost on my fellow passengers nor me as we vigorously made our collective concerns abundantly clear to our faltering Herman.

His empty, wispy reassurances and extended, increasingly sporadic bursts on the burner did nothing to ease anyone's nerves, or the balloon's trajectory.

If anything, we seemed to gather speed until seconds from impact, Herman, in a thick accent, bellowed, 'Brace yourselves!' We clattered into, uprooted, and dragged the only tree as far as the eye could see 10-metres across the heathland. The landing had been so hard, it had thrown the basket on its side and had its younger occupants clambering out on all fours, while the old woman, crumpled and groaning, had been saved by the cushioning bodies of the old couple. Once the son and I had retrieved his mother and had her standing, shaking uncontrollably, I looked around at the excited faces from earlier. The young, couple were embracing, crying on each other's shoulder, the older gentleman had lost his pair of binoculars and ripped his shirt, and my girlfriend stood in shock, trying to locate one of her leather boots that had come off during the near-fatal landing. The bent, bright brass memorial plaque attached to the buckled, black cage confirmed its recent planting and did nothing to lighten the group's mood.

While we were still coming to terms with our near-death experiences, the Red Baron had swiftly radioed in and been picked up and driven away in a Land Rover, leaving his team to pack away the balloon and us waiting for a minibus of unknown whereabouts.

It hadn't been the romantic morning we had hoped for and in much the same way the balloon had come crashing down, so did the relationship shortly after.

Single again, I floundered around trying to find a job that didn't lead to a mental breakdown. It was during one of my many internet searches that I first stumbled across the psychological condition, 'Boarding School Syndrome'. Before you start thinking poor rich kid and stop reading, let me try and explain. Those that read *Lady Luck and Me* will know about my childhood or more specifically, my schooling. For those that haven't, in a nutshell, I was sent to a boarding school before I'd reached double figures whilst my mother and new-step father moved to Germany on an army posting. It would be months before I would see my mother again and when other boarders went home for weekends and half-terms I would be at school on my own, feeding myself with whatever I could find in the school kitchen and then putting myself to bed after I'd scared myself stupid watching inappropriately adult films late on channel 4. Occasionally, certain teacher's unknown to mother and step-father would bath me at weekends. Homesickness cried me to sleep most nights.

When I did go home, I had my travel documents in a bright orange pouch that hung around my neck. I held hands with a Lufthansa employee as they chaperoned me around the airport and onto the plane. Aside from my prick step-father, 'Barrie the bastard', who made home-life miserable, there was a boy of similar age who lived opposite and schooled locally, Rupert King-Evans, that used to taunt me that parents only sent their children to boarding schools because they didn't want them. It was a very convincing argument at that age and one that I had no evidence to prove otherwise. At the end of each home visit, I tried everything I could muster to stay but nothing ever worked and when I was taken by the hand by another Lufthansa employee with my travel documents swinging in its orange pouch, I would hurt my neck, twisting it so I could see my mother for as long as I could before the doors closed, knowing it would months until I saw her face again. I was at boarding school until the age of 18 and would have gladly traded all the so-called 'privileges' of private school for the love or company of family and friends, and a sense of wanted belonging.

Anyway, when I read about 'Boarding School Syndrome', seismic pieces of my mental ill-health puzzle fell into place. Abandonment and separation fears, sense of failure, low self-esteem, depression, anxiety, isolation, trust and commitment issues. The diagnosis eased the long-held belief that I was uniquely broken. Although I found comfort in discovering a condition that defined many of my problems, it was no cure.

O FATHER, MY FATHER

'It's all a reasonable child can expect if the dad is present at the conception.' – **Joe Orton**

DESPITE THIS PSYCHOLOGICAL revelation, I was no further along in establishing a career with healthy longevity. My searches ranged vastly and increasingly desperate. From joining the French foreign legion to belly-dancing classes in Azerbaijan, nothing was off the table. One advertisement that popped up was for qualified, close protection officers (bodyguards), needed both domestically and abroad. Being single, with no dependants and rock bottom self-esteem, it sounded perfect, but first, I needed the qualification.

There are several training facilities dotted around the world, including the industry-respected 'Ronin' in South Africa, where, for five weeks and around £6000, you learn everything required to be a fully-fledged CPO from ex-special forces personnel. Included in the package were evasive driving techniques, weapons training, hand-to-hand combat, and tasering both someone else and yourself.

My father, who was still trying to make his millions from one end of a bar, was beside himself when he heard my plans. I think he always saw himself as a henchman, so he took great pride in telling his wealthier, impressionable friends that violence ran in the blood. He was busy setting up Ugandan Airways from his sleepy pub in West Sussex and, being the realistic person and doting father he is, informally asked whether I would go to Kampala as head of the airline's security. I'd be responsible for recruitment, training, risk assessment, etc., while he would remain at HQ, Guinness in hand. I reminded him that I'd been a brief, useless salesman and a bookshop employee for the previous five years, and my stint as a Muay Thai fighter hardly qualified me as a suitable candidate. Also, as a director of this multi-million venture, his reluctance to leave his place of business and visit the venue threw familiar red flags all over the place.

After cursory consideration, I thanked him for his thoughtful and generous offer but decided it wasn't quite the right fit for me. Nonetheless, I continued scratching my head for ways to pay for the course when my father introduced me to one of his 'work' associates, 'Big Nick.' And 'Big Nick' was big, in length rather than width, in his fifties with a killer deep voice and connections to people in the CPO industry. He was a wealth of dark art knowledge, having lived experience in various security and CPO scenarios around the world.

When father left us to recharge his glass, 'Big Nick' asked for my thoughts on a simple, one-way, A-B contract off the West African coast. Application requirements were vague, which usually attracted nefarious mercenaries and private security firms, but as no formal qualification was necessary, anyone with or without a brain could apply. Terms and conditions weren't discussed, but with a nod and a wink, he implied that it would be an attractive package. I told him I needed time to consider doing one of the most senseless things in my life and would be sure to be in touch if I wanted further details.

A few days later, I received a text message from my father. He was at 'work' and had been chatting to 'Big Nick' about my interest in the West African contract and had kindly taken it upon himself to be the broker of any future dealings, meaning all communication should go directly through him.

All the years of healing and careful trust-building, gone. That was the end of my relationship with my father. It was another reminder not to get too close, too attached and not to trust. Several years later, I received an email from him, asking to rekindle our relationship and being utterly confounded as to why communication had abruptly stopped in the first place. His lifelong mantra of 'people are currency' clearly knows no bounds and so, to this day, he is no longer referred to as Colin but Colon.

I politely declined 'Big Nicks's' invitation to put my name forward, preferring to make a living on dry land, away from crazed, twitchy-fingered pirates and their loaded AK-47's and as the months crept by, my interest in paying to be tasered and then taking a bullet for a wealthy, dickhead stranger, slowly waned.

ANTON

'I love the deep conversations your eyes have with mine'
– John Mark Green

With no job prospects and a mistrustful father who would sell me for half a pint of Guinness, my mental health started to decline again. My black dog always returns to feed when I lose direction and hope, and I had lost both. I began to socially withdraw further and further, preferring to stare at the tree tops from my bedroom window for hours than seek out company. The shortening of the days didn't help. Grey, dead unremarkable days drifted into forgettable weeks, robbing the last of any residual will. During particularly challenging episodes, the three yards from my bed to the bathroom became impossible and had me reach for anything that could hold my urine. My years of reliable, numbing medication were faltering, as was my confidence in leaving my room. For weeks, I could be in a paralysed limbo between not wanting to be dead and not wanting to be alive either.

When I was unfit to leave my room, I switched off all modes of communication. The phone was allowed to die; the laptop left to gather dust, even the TV was largely ignored. In the rare moments when I had the mental strength to power up my phone, I would often regret it. There would be no messages or missed calls many days after going dark, reinforcing the thought that I wasn't being missed by the world or anyone in it. When times became very bleak, I would repetitively stab the top of my left arm with anything sharp enough to make blood pour in torrents down the arm. The frantic action would spray the white walls with thin, spotty red lines, making the room look like a Jackson Pollock studio. I would cry hard, ashamed of what I was doing, the need for what I was doing, for being a disappointment, lonely, broken, and born. Self-harm is never to be condoned, but I can absolutely understand the assumed benefits of historic blood-letting which dates back over 3000 years to the ancient Egyptians. For me, it was cathartic. It was a purging, a release of the inner scream, albeit temporary but being non-committal in ending myself permanently, it was the next best therapeutic relief.

On stronger days, aside from my mother, the only other person I would contemplate leaving my room for was our next-door neighbour, Debbie. I only seem to know women called Debbie. Despite our friendship, both households had mutual respect for privacy, but on good evenings when we saw her, she brought nothing but unbridled joy and rib-tickling laughter. From trying to home the bearded lady of Guildford to rehoming a wingless turkey in Turkey, her heart knows no bounds. She's one of the kindest, most compassionate people I know.

Nearing the conclusion of one of our evenings the discussion moved onto mental health and the doubtless, countless benefits of regular, outdoor exercise. For me, doing exercise simply because it was good for my mental health would never be strong enough motivation for when I was unable to leave my room and pissing in bottles, but having something I valued more than myself just might be the difference. An hour later, a photo of a nearly Labrador, golden in colour with a pink nose, dropped through the letterbox. On the reverse side was written, 'Anton.'

Anton was in Malaga, Spain, residing in an outdoor, stony pen, having been removed from the city streets by the local council's dog warden 18 months previously. The English charity that was keeping him only had limited time and even more limited resources, and both were rapidly depleting, as were his days wandering this earth. We hadn't considered getting a dog, especially another rescue, and contrary to the advice of the nearest and dearest, we began making earnest inquiries.

We were assured that he was a gentle soul, about two years old, and had successfully passed the all-important cat test. They didn't share any details on how the cat test was carried out, which made me wonder what constituted a fail and whether they used the same cat each time. Adopting a dog from Spain must be nearly as complicated as adopting Siamese twins from Mars. The paperwork alone is monstrous. Reams of the stuff flooded through the letterbox, asking every imaginable question. What was your first pet called? Do you like the film 'Babe'? Have you watched 'Lassie'? We also had three scheduled and one unannounced home visit from the charity's English contingent, checking criminal records and our home's suitability. Once all the hurdles had been jumped and his vaccinations, passport, and transport fees had been administered and paid, we waited for his arrival.

It took the white panel van three days to reach us, it's first stop. Some of the other unfortunate occupants were heading to North Yorkshire and Scotland, at least another day's drive, meaning some dogs would be in windowless transit for four or five days. Representatives of the charity had arranged to be present for the off-loading, so there were four of us standing in nervous silence by the front door when the van pulled up and two men got out. Conditions in the back of the van looked grim, and the stench matched it. Cages on cages of furry faces with black, terrified eyes peered out. It was miserable to witness. According to the driver, he had given them all a brief leg-stretch on entering the country an hour earlier, although Anton's wonky stumble suggested otherwise. With his tail tucked tightly between his legs, he was slowly and reluctantly led trembling to us. Once inside, he pissed twice and tried his best to hide behind the living room curtains for the first two hours.

According to his passport, Anton was part Labrador, part Spinone (Italian hunting dog), and polydactyl. I thought Polydactyly's had died out in the Jurassic age but on our inaugural visit to the vets, was gleefully informed that it simply meant that he had defunct, dangling hindleg dewclaws that only become a problem if they get caught, which of course, they did. The vet's excitement at making an easy, fat buck was short-lived when we discovered Anton's four Achilles heels are, well, his four heels. For all his placid qualities, he won't let anyone go within a foot of his feet, let alone handle them. He goes from 0-200 within a blink of an eye and if his jaws don't get you, the shock of his movement makes your heart skip a beat, a sensation the vet experienced repeatedly. They tried sedatives in his food, in his water, darkened rooms until, finally, a tranquiliser dart sent him reluctantly to sleep. (On a side note, I want to thank all the gods for the marvellous Petplan. Without them, my mother and I would have had to have sold both kidneys for just walking through the door.)

Anton is, without question, the campest dog I've ever known. His go-to prone position is with his two front paws crossed, with a peculiar, as my sister calls it, 'porn look' on his face, much to everyone's amusement. If he had opposable thumbs, the first thing he would do is knit a rainbow frock. He's also one of only two Anton's I've ever met, the other being none other than twinkle toes himself, Anton Du Beke, and due to a strange twist of fate, the two Anton's have crossed paths. It was on a mundane Tuesday afternoon. Anton (four-legged) and I had popped into the empty local to take my usual place at the end of the bar, pen and paper in hand, nearest the comforting, crackling log fire. Half a pint in, with my mind in neutral, the door opened and in floated Mr. Du Beke and his then-dance partner, 'Honey,' from Eastenders. We all politely acknowledged each other before they decided upon a table by the window in the corner. 'Honey,' being a parish resident and fellow dog-lover, saw Anton with his paws crossed, 'porn face' on, giggled, and came over to say hello.

Her face lit up when she heard his name and immediately beckoned over Mr. Du Beke. While he glided effortlessly through the tables, Anton the hound majestically rose and tip-tapped his long claws across the wooden floor like Fred Astaire, where the couple met in the middle. For the first time ever, Anton held up his limp right paw to be regally shaken, and shaken it was, with vigour. When Mr. Du Beke crouched to eye level, there was an almost tangible 'Anton' brotherhood, cross-species connection. While 'Honey' and I made awkward, small talk about 'Dirty Den,' the Anton's gazed into each other eyes for a little too long for comfort. I can safely say, 'Honey' and I both felt a pang of jealousy of our respective partners as they shared their moment. Alas, sadly, all good things must end, so when my dazzling conversation with 'Honey' was interrupted by the barman, and before the Anton's could book a room, the two were forced apart with the sadness of a Shakespearean tragedy. I can't be sure, but when Mr. Du Beke turned for his table, it looked very much like he wiped something from the corner of his eye.

My Anton has been a life-saver, and I don't say that glibly. Without him in my life and if I was breathing, and that's a big if, I would have regressed into being a fulltime bed-bound hermit. He is indeed the gentlest of souls, my closest advisor and my best friend.

I WILL BREAK YOU

'She dresses to the left.' – **Patrick Murray**

ON THE HEALTHY days between episodes, I was taking more and more of a macabre interest at the alarming, exponential upward trend of male suicides. Having myself so nearly been a statistic many times and always been left wanting at the lack of accessible services open specifically to men, I thought I had to at least try something. So, with another friend who had also been through similar struggles and shared similar concerns, 'The League of Unextraordinary Gentlemen' was born.

Grammatically, our name didn't make sense, but neither did we. Both single, both in our early 40's, both unemployed and both disillusioned with life. Our objective was clear, and our mission statement was simple; reach out to other struggling men and organise local events where they can speak openly to others without fear of judgment.

First, we needed to market our not-for-profit enterprise, and after an extensive social media marketing campaign, our numbers swelled to four. Tee shirts were printed and freely distributed to our small band of broken brothers, and once a week, we would meet at the recreation ground for an hour of general fitness before heading to the pub until last orders.

To raise awareness and funds for more tee shirts and another successful social media campaign, I arranged a drag night in 'The Star', Godalming on a Friday night. Fliers were flown, posters were pinned, and our marketing juggernaut was revved up and let loose once again. Jules, an old friend, fashion writer, and experienced drag show attendee, was invited from London on the promise of a night to remember. As the date neared, even I was slightly surprised by the positive interest shown by pub patrons and geared-up for the avalanche of tee-shirt orders.

Being the organiser, it was only fitting to fully commit to the evening and therefore, after considerable thought, decided to transform myself into Yoshiko, the Japanese Geisha. The local party shop supplied the necessary attire, and having slipped into her robes like I felt I had a thousand times before, began on her make-up. An hour and a half later, I started to regret my decision to go as the beautiful Yoshiko. The thick, white foundation did nothing to hide my protruding stubble, and no matter how hard I concentrated on getting the lipstick right, I couldn't escape looking like a freakish clown. It was questionable whether my choice could be deemed politically correct, maybe even racist, but as I stared at myself in the mirror, it was bitter-sweet to acknowledge that I looked so shit, I couldn't possibly offend anyone, apart from clowns. Meanwhile, my dear 6'4" friend, Ian, happily married with two children, was having his own struggles getting into a pair of nude high heels, all the while trying to stop his blonde wig from getting caught in his false, spider-leg eyelashes every time he refined his hair flick.

While I nervously tottered the short distance to the pub in my floral pencil dress with painted toenails in geta footwear, Ian cat-walked in his 'little black dress' with such assurance and elegance, I found it wholly unbelievable to hear that was his first outing as 'Michelle from the East end'. His subtle wig corrections in shop windows and the speed and grace at which he moved over the uneven cobbles in his heels was something to stand by and admire. As I shouldered a burdening feeling of regret, Ian, by his own admission, 'felt amazing'.

The pub was rammed, rammed like I'd never seen before. I was heartened, even moved by such a positive response. While we stood on the pavement waiting for entry, I couldn't help thinking how glad I was that we had decided to cancel our appalling rendition of 'Yes sir, I can boogie'. Meanwhile, Ian blushed and simpered meekly at two wolf whistles from passing cars before yet again readjusting his hair and reapplying more lipstick in his compact mirror, which his ruby red nail-painted fingers had delicately plucked from a silver-chained, black sequined clutch handbag.

Once we were in, it became immediately evident why it was so exceptionally busy. The pub, for the first time ever, was hosting a touring, drunk rugby team from Huddersfield, and sitting at the end of the bar, fighting off stranger's hairy hands, Eric. Eric was 'The League of Unextraordinary Gentleman's' third recruit. He's a small, handsome, shy man; with an undiscovered talent for applying make-up it seemed. Perched daintily on a bar stool, wearing a feather boa, tiny mini-skirt, and stockings, he was convincing as he was awkward, not daring to raise his gaze above his flute of prosecco. He was also the only person in a packed pub of about 150 who had supported the cause. Considering that we were trying to reach out to struggling men, particularly those suffering from anxiety, low self-esteem, and low confidence, attracting everyone's attention by wearing drag probably wasn't the wisest way to promote a stress-free mental health group. Contrastingly, Ian worked the crowded pub with uncanny ease, trailing Eric's feather boa across as many shoulders as he could and flicking his hair around as if he was auditioning for a part in Footloose.

I sat with Eric at the bar, offering protection and my heartfelt condolences as he held back the tears. After a while, the rugby team got tired of groping Eric in favour of the far more accommodating Ian, leaving us staring at our drinks in traumatic silence. I think the third Sambuca broke Eric, sending him home quietly sobbing, not before he had slurred to me it had been his worst night ever. I felt entirely responsible. By the time Jules arrived from London, I was a drunken, emotional mess that had somehow lost my right geta and had ripped my pencil dress up to my thigh. Ian however, glowed and was now doing his best to convince me to go to the only bar in town with a late licence, but more importantly to Ian and his new rugby friends, a dancefloor.

There was no way I was going anywhere to dance, so when Ian phoned his wife for a lift home, Jules poured me into a taxi home, much in the same state as Eric had left a few forgotten hours earlier.

Maybe not surprisingly, we didn't receive a single inquiry regarding 'The League of Unextraordinary Gentlemen' or take any tee-shirt orders. In fact, the only anonymous email queried Eric's upcoming availability. If anything, the night had done far more damage than good, wounding some more deeply than others. On the plus side, Ian, who was beaming from ear to ear when I saw him the following Monday evening enthusiastically asked,

'Mate, I had such a good night. When can we do that again?'

Over the next few months, interest in 'The League of Unextraordinary Gentlemen' slowly diminished until I was the only one wearing the tee shirt. Despite its colossal failure, it had, in its brief existence, given me a worthwhile purpose and a rare sense of usefulness, so much so and without a whiff of any other options or ideas, started looking for any possibility of a making a living within the mental health sector. With decades of experience but no formal qualifications, my search returned very few results. All paths required training, but I neither had the financial resources nor appetite to return to university for three years, so instead, looked for other accessible avenues into the industry, which led to me to 'Mental Health First Aid England' and their instructor course.

The course was held in central London and was attended by 15 from all over the country. Many belonged to housing associations and were there under their respective employee's duress and against their will, which they demonstrated with total disinterest from the outset. Some wore earphones, while others feared separation anxiety, refusing to put their phone down, even during the role-playing exercises. The few of us that were there independently and had paid a pretty penny for the privilege were less than impressed. One of them, a lady in her fifties who had travelled down from Durham, had had enough by day three and discharged both barrels at a chap in his thirties for his loud outbursts as he watched live horse racing on his phone.

The course itself was broken into two categories. The first two days were spent doing the first aid course, and the following three days were spent on how to deliver that first aid course. At the end, students were assessed on their presentation skills, with successful graduates invited to join their membership. It was a helpful course, albeit slightly basic but genuinely educational. Underpinning it all was the clear message that we were not there to 'fix' people's mental health but to give them valuable tools to deal with any future crisis. My suspicions that money was a higher priority than their compassion was first raised when everyone on the course passed, even the girl who had fallen asleep during the slideshow of her own presentation.

Another questionable aspect was that all materials, including stationary, had to be exclusively supplied by them at full price. Considering each course book cost £20 per student, plus the other add-ons, which had to be paid upfront, the outlay to the instructor was considerable, resulting in profit margins being very lean indeed.

My one and only course was co-instructed with Kay, who had spent hours organising a conference room in London, for two days for 12 people. There was a fair amount of confusion at the beginning when I had to source a 13th chair. We all introduced ourselves, apart from one man in his forties who sat silently smiling at everyone around him. It took us nearly half an hour to establish he was supposed to be in the conference room above, attending the 'Introduction to the English language: Stage 1' course.

The 12 attendees all came from different backgrounds and all had their reasons for being there. Many told desperately sad personal stories and sought answers, understanding, and peace. At times, it was challenging to listen to. The virgin box of tissues that was passed around took an hour to empty.

By the end of the second day, I was emotionally exhausted. It had been far more harrowing than I had foreseen and had triggered many of my own deeply buried memories and insecurities. Once I had deducted the travel expenses, the books, stationery costs, and half the conference room, I was left with just enough money to buy a bottle of wine to soften some of the awful tragedies I had heard and rebury some of my own.

A couple of weeks later, the instructors were invited to Canary Wharf, where upper management would outline their vision for the coming year and listen to instructor's concerns and suggestions. The organisers had vastly underestimated the number of attendees and went about hastily acquiring additional seating from other conference rooms while issuing thanks for people's patience. As the instructors hopped from foot to foot in discomfort, the front two rows had been roped off for management and various spurious VIPs. Whilst we waited, they flitted about triple kissing each other and laughing so artificially it was like a pretentious Hollywood cocktail party. After the fourth request, the final VIP took her seat, only to be immediately invited onto the stage where as a founder, she cooed that she couldn't be prouder of what they had achieved in the past year. Every breath and deliberate pause in her forty-minute list of achievements was greeted with exuberant applause from the two front rows. The speaker revelled in their congratulations, taking obvious pleasure in dampening their enthusiasm by occasionally raising her hand. Three others spoke from the front row, all heaping heavy, sycophantic praise on each other and another tremendous year. The rest of us, some sitting but most still standing, looked on in silence, with growing irritated bemusement. When the last speaker had finally finished and sat down to yet another extended round of applause, a serious-looking young woman with long dark hair and a headset escorted the two front rows of back-slapping VIP's out of the room. Only when the last, with the loudest cackle had filed out of the room did another head-set wearing organiser appear on the stage to tell the rest of us we were welcome to enjoy a tea break. However, it would be on a first-come, first-served basis as they had neither the crockery nor biscuits to accommodate everyone.

Returning from the empty tea table, I re-joined the more able instructors standing at the back of the room and awaited the VIP's reappearance. Not a single chair had been taken when an aging lady in an ankle-length, green sequinned dress, heavy foundation and lip-sticked teeth took to the stage with a wireless microphone in hand. Trailing behind her was one of the hairiest and most rotund men I've ever seen, wearing a sweat-stained, thinning, faded Metallica tee-shirt, open-toed Jesus sandals with lank, long greasy hair that got caught in his beard. Huffing and puffing, he pushed a small squeaky trolley that had a beginner's electric keyboard, a speaker and a disco ball to the front and parked it next to the raised platform. We stood and sat there, watching as they struggled to untangle bundles of leads and then carry out a full 5-minute sound check. I've never heard, 'testing, testing 1…2, testing, testing, testing 1…2…3, testing' so very many times.

When they were finally ready, the volume of her introductions made the floor vibrate and people cover their ears. Introductions over, she asked the mystified audience to stand, and then signalled to her keyboard companion. He solemnly nodded as if he was conducting a funeral service and pressed a beat button on the keyboard. As she lost herself in her own appalling interpretation of Desperado, he encouraged the audience to follow him in clapping along. It was a poor, inappropriate choice, terribly performed. She was so woefully flat people winced. The beat sounded like it had been borrowed from a German trance nightclub, and the lone multicoloured disco light on the trolley had already stopped roaming the room and was now going through its range of colours on the crotch of the keyboard player. They were the kind of double act that entertained care homes residents between bingo games.

Her theatrical bow at the end of Desperado was met with a smattering of half-hearted applause. To her credit, she didn't take all the praise, she turned to her profusely sweating keyboard player and clapped him as he took an unwarranted bow. Asking us to remain standing, not that most of us had a choice, she divided the room down the central aisle into two. Another signal to the keyboard player and another beat button was pushed. This time, she started bellowing out Coldplay's 'Fix you', pointing to one side of the room and then the other to echo her every time she said 'fix you'. One lady to the right started but immediately fell silent as the rest of the room stood in utter disbelief at what they were witnessing. They were oblivious, both lost in their glorious, imaginary rockstar worlds.

I was one of the last to leave, transfixed by the irony of the situation and wondering what other faux pas they had up their sleeves. I could still hear her warbling away when the lift doors opened on the ground level, two floors below.

Considering the whole day had come out of our own pockets, I found the entire experience gross. The outrageous self-congratulatory platitudes grated. There was no mention of their vision for the following year, and absolutely nothing was spoken about the people we were there to help or mental health in general. I vowed then and there that they wouldn't be getting any more of my rapidly lessening finances.

It had also been the defining moment for Kay to start looking elsewhere for employment. We said our goodbyes and went our separate ways, although that wasn't the last I saw of Kay. A month later, I watched her on 'The Chase,' getting through the first round but failing to take any money home, and then two weeks later, on 'Tipping Point,' again sadly leaving empty-handed. It's a risky strategy to make a living, but it's better than funding those pompous dickheads and the world's worst two musicians.

SHERLOCK HOLMOSEXUAL

'Coo-ee! Any homo? – **Harry Enfield**

HAVING DECIDED AGAINST life as a 'Mental Health First Aid Instructor' and a professional gunslinger, I turned my hand to the gentler alternative of researching and writing about the relatively unknown but fascinating town of Godalming. '*Oh my Godalming*' was terrible and a regret. Not only was it poorly researched, poorly written, and briskly published, but I recklessly threw trusted friends 'under the bus' for cheap shits and giggles. My feeble attempts at distorting distinguishing details were, at best, transparent and, at worst, downright insulting. If anything, my changes only succeeded in publicly portraying the easily recognisable local characters and my friends as privileged narcissists. I understand and deserve the resulting ostracism.

But aside from demonising people and losing friends, I did discover some wacky and wonderful facts about the town that once boasted '*the best overall quality of life in the country*' – *Telegraph newspaper, March 2013*

For a start, it was the first town in the world to install electric street lighting. Yes indeed. A pioneer for the world over. Jack Phillips, the chief wireless telegraphist of the doomed Titanic, and hero for repeatedly sending SOS messages as the ship went down, once called it home. But for me, Godalming's most outstanding historical resident must surely go to a 25-year-old, married, illiterate servant, Mary Toft.

In September 1726, Mary made national headline news for giving birth to a collection of eye-watering objects. These included legs of a cat, a hog's bladder, and 18 dead rabbits. Let me repeat that: a cat's legs, a hog's bladder, and 18 dead rabbits. So bizarre was her case that King George I, who was on the throne at the time, dispatched his head surgeon to investigate. After witnessing a stillborn rabbit birth first-hand, he confirmed Mary's case to be legitimate and valid and transported her to London for further probing. When threatened with a painful internal examination, Mary declared the whole affair a hoax, revealing that a porter had been paid to source the 'ingredients,' which she then inserted into herself before delivering them.

Consequently, she was jailed for being '*a notorious and vile cheat*' while the embarrassed medical practitioners became the laughing stock of the country. She was briefly revered for being a witch by some, although she wasn't being accused of pulling rabbits out of a hat. Mary returned to Godalming no richer or brighter than when she had left and carried on her life in relative obscurity, occasionally being hired by wealthy individuals to 'entertain' guests at dinner parties.

While discovering how others scratched a living in the 18th century, I was scratching my head. Unfortunately, my anatomy didn't allow me to follow in Mary's footsteps, even if I did think I would be a natural. As it happens, my following line of work came from an unusual source.

One regular at the local pub, Clive, was a quiet chap in his 50s, always with a book underarm, who kept himself to himself, supping and reading. Over time, Clive and I began talking, usually about whatever he was reading, and then as the relationship developed, broader aspects of life. The pigeon-holing of where you live, what you do, and what car you drive were all refreshingly absent. Eventually, albeit reluctantly, it came to light that he was a private investigator. When I thought of private investigators, I pictured Hawaiian shirts, red Ferraris, and moustaches so splendid they could tickle a fanny from five hundred yards. He ticked nor tickled any of those boxes. He stood 5'5" at best, wore a faded, baggy, black leather jacket, oversized ragged jeans, and worn black leather shoes; drove a non-descript family estate car, and had a top lip as smooth as a baby baboon's bottom. None of this transpired by accident, except for his height. In his profession, it's good field craft to be as unremarkable as possible and he did it magnificently. He never discussed cases and never disclosed names or places. I found his integrity astonishing.

One summer evening, he told me he was looking for someone to help him out for the day. I loved the idea of carrying out surveillance or springing a honey trap on a bastard husband, so I jumped at the chance. It turned out it was none of the above. I was to be paid a cool £100 a day to walk around more exhibition halls and point interested parties to our stand, but this time with a fake, plastic monocle, smoking a fake pipe, wearing a cheap, ill-fitting, polyester Sherlock Holmes costume that had been clearly designed for swinger's parties and seedy strip joints. I looked like a total bell-end.

The first expo was at a local racecourse, midweek. The 'hall' was about the size of a double-garage with our stand alone taking up 1\4 of the room. The three other exhibitors were a microbrewery, a local butcher, and an under 9s homemade cake stand, raising money for a Romanian donkey sanctuary. It wasn't the demographic he had hoped. Unsurprisingly, none of the seven parents that attended required his services and he dismissed the whole experience as pointless. Not to me, however. It was an easy £100, and for that money, I didn't mind looking like a misplaced, cross-dressing stripper for the day.

The next expo was the other end of the spectrum. Determined to generate new, relevant leads, he booked a stand at a law convention at the Excel in London. This time our stand was dwarfed by multi-national companies such as KPMG, Pricewaterhousecoopers, Dentons and was healthily attended by thousands, all expensively suited and booted. As I obediently wandered the aisles, trying to get visitors to our stand, I was dying inside. Rightfully, I was viewed as a novelty, with people queuing to take their photos with me; some even gave me small donations. As the blisters grew, so did the Stuttgart flashbacks. I couldn't wait for the day to end. To some aspiring actors, this would be a fun day to make £100, but as an introvert when sober, I found it deeply deflating. I had grossly underestimated the scale of the event and hadn't expected to be routinely laughed at for 8 hours. Every camera click felt like a punch to the stomach.

Meanwhile, in the absence of visitors to our stand, Clive had been busy watching people gather around the opposite stand, trying their luck at the combination code of a safe that secured a £500 Amazon voucher. After a brief conversation with the two lady exhibitors, it transpired out that no one had ever managed to crack it since its inception over 50 shows ago. They even joked that they had forgotten the combination. When the doors closed at the end of the day and holders were beginning to dismantle their stands, Clive casually wandered over, gained their permission to have a go, and on the first attempt, opened the 4" reinforced steel door, retrieved the voucher, shut the door and wished them a pleasant evening. They were speechless, then absolutely livid, and began by telling him he didn't qualify and that only members of the paying public were eligible. His composed, silent smile did nothing to help. They then accused him of being a con man trickster and threatened to call the police if he didn't return it, which was met with the same dismissive silence. He was a wise, old owl who had dealt with more significant threats in his shady career than two middle-aged, overweight women waving their fingers at him.

I'd never been happier to hand back a stripper's outfit than I was that evening, and while I left with my pride in tatters and yet another gaping hole in my heel, Clive was reasonably chuffed with his day's work. He never answered my questions on how he managed it and to this day, it still remains a mystery.

Impersonating Sherlock Holmes had been an unmitigated disaster, but the life of a P.I. intrigued me, so much so that I enrolled in an online P.I diploma course and began growing an ugly slug under my nose. During my studies, I spent a couple of days a week in Clive's remote office, following up on inquiries and getting a better feel for what the role entailed. There were three of us in the office; Clive, myself, and an attractive girl in her 20s who did office admin and the honey-trapping. Occasionally, another P.I. based in Southampton would visit. He was a married man in his forties, had two young children, and was a regular, likeable, straightforward family man for all intents and purposes. Or that was what I thought.

One unremarkable day I was at my computer working my way through contact lists when Clive summoned me to an adjoining meeting room where the Southampton P.I was rigidly sitting at the table. It was the first time the three of us had been together, so as the door was closed behind me, I was excited to hear about my part in their scheming. Sitting opposite the Southampton P.I., with pen and paper at the ready, Clive asked me the least expected, most unusual question.

'Would you sleep with him?'

I let out an uncomfortable giggle and looked at them both thinking it was a joke I hadn't understood. Without a hint of sarcasm, the question was repeated.

'Would *you* sleep with *him*?'

The P.I. opposite sat oddly motionless, fists clenched, staring at the table in front of him, while Clive peered at me, waiting for an answer. I'm a happily heterosexual man and wouldn't go near him even if his dick had been double-dipped in diamonds. As I sat there confused, it suddenly dawned on me that I had been used as an unwitting honey trap all along. It all made sense; the befriending, the alluring stripper's outfit. Clive had played me like a piano.

'Go fuck yourselves!' was as polite as I could muster at the time, and with that, I was up and off, slamming every door behind me as I went, never to return and permanently terminating our faux friendship.

Since I had paid for my course, I decided to complete it, but this latest surreal episode made me question the morality and ethics of the people who worked in the industry. And so there ended my dreams of becoming a modern-day Sherlock Holmes. The adolescent slug was removed, the Hawaiian shirts returned, and the Ferrari would just have to wait for another day.

HANDICAPS

'Golf is not a sport, it's a career move' – **Rachel Bradley, Cold Feet**

DETERMINED NEVER TO set foot inside another exhibition hall again or to wear such sexy, provocative stripper's clothing so well, my next employment strategy led me to Guildford Job Centre. Having qualified over two decades ago in Sports Science with Business Management, I'm almost exclusively certified to be a leisure centre manager or a bowling alley shoe-man, so as the months rolled by, it came as no surprise that very few relevant opportunities arose.

Once a month, I would pilgrimage to see my case worker, who would talk me through various unrealistic positions, gently quiz me on my work efforts and then authorize my monthly Jobseekers Allowance as it was back then.

One month, however, that changed.

Having walked the route so many times previously, I was on autopilot. With my headphones in, staring at my feet, I completely failed to notice the young Japanese couple in front of me abruptly stop midway across the road to take a selfie in front of a church. The first I knew of it was my heavy landing on the two-wheeled case she was dragging behind her. Thankfully it broke my fall. Not so thankfully, it broke the case, the handle of the case and very nearly her delicate arm. Going to her aid, I was angrily shoed away, literally shoed away with a dangerous-looking high heel, as he tried stuffing her clothes back into the knackered case. Unsure of what to do, I stood around like a lemon profusely apologising while he shoved pants into his pocket, and she held her porcelain arm, staring at her smashed iPhone screen.

The angry, fat, white-van man in a stained vest that came at me and 'politely' requested I make my way off the road and to the pavement was actually most welcome. In his haste, the poor Japanese man stuffed what he could into the case, crammed it shut, thrust it under his arm, took his girlfriend's limp hand, and ran off the crossing the way they had come, leaving a single yellow trainer, a pair of rolled socks and two crumpled shirts stranded behind. By the time I had reached the safety of the opposite pavement, the white-van man had returned to his mechanical steed and seemed to take great gratification in lining up the trainer and making sure both front and rear wheels made contact before giving me 'the bird' and reminding me that I'm a 'wanker'. Unusual as it sounds, I must applaud that odious little man. Without his impassioned, romantically worded intervention, there's a slim chance I would have presented at A & E with bizarre, borderline believable shoe injuries.

Arriving at the jobcentre, I was surprised to see my case worker standing at the top of the stairs, grinning from ear to ear like a submariner in a brothel. On reaching his desk, he enthusiastically informed me that he had the perfect job. Naturally, I immediately enquired whether it was exhibition-related, stripper-related, or envelope-related, and when I was comforted that it was none of them, took a seat.

He nearly burst telling me that my local golf club was looking for an assistant golf pro. I had worked in a golf club 25 years ago as a part-time waiter and had watched the pro fill his time putting balls around the quiet shop. I could do that. I'd watched the Ryder cup highlights. Times were hard, and a job's a job after all. Despite never having had a handicap or owned a glove, I applied.

A week later, I was shifting uncomfortably in a chair in front of the general manager, singing the praises of Ping clubs and laughing at bogus tales of my time playing in the Far East.

Unbelievably, I'd done enough. When I arrived home, there was a message on the answering machine congratulating me on my new appointment and asking me to start the following Monday.

I owned one club, my grandfather's bamboo shafted putter, and one old cracked driving range ball and had neither the money to invest in more clubs, the time to research golf, nor the talent required for a handicap. I did buy a glove though. An expensive leather one that looked great hanging out of my chino's back pocket.

My first day in the shop with the pro involved a lot of chin-stroking, a lot of toilet breaks, and unavoidable comparisons of each other's choice of clubs, players, and techniques. Initially, I spent most of my time in the shop, on the phone, booking tee times, and selling Mars bars while the pro taught lessons. The retail side was fine, I had a card-reader and a float this time, but I was seriously out of my depth in any coaching capacity. Occasionally, I would be asked for my thoughts from members on clubs, clothes, and their swing. Once I had colour coordinated them from head to foot, their confidence in me foolishly grew. All technique advice involved them standing before me and showing me their swing. More chin stroking would inevitably follow as I searched for the relevant, golfing lingo. My go-to instruction of minutely adjusting their grip usually sufficed. For the stubborn, suspicious minority, I insisted on seeing them on the course, hitting a ball before advising on any profound technical improvements, safe in the knowledge it would never happen.

As I was getting more familiar with the members and starting to believe that I could actually pull this off, the club steward invited me along to talk through the course. Off we went side by side in an official buggy. He was a keen golfer, long-term member and knew the course like the back of his retired hand. His formal questioning on how I would approach a green, whether I would fade off a tee and which club I'd use where and my woolly, inadequate answers left me sure I'd be back at the job centre within a week. Surprisingly, I was back in the shop the next day, selling retirees thousand-pound sets of golf clubs, waterproof trousers, and the promise of a better game. The slight technical adjustments I'd nervously offered initially were growing into a complete technique overhaul.

One lady member, who had a handicap of 9, was so desperate to improve her game that she was willing to listen and fund any new idea. I vividly recall her telling me that she thought my shopfloor theories were 'unorthodox,' but, as I was twenty years her junior and had played in the Far East recently, she was open to suggestions and booked me. Within a month, I had gone from being unable to pronounce 'Titleist' to charging my first client £25 an hour.

Still having been unable to invest in any clubs, I borrowed a member's set that had been brought in to the shop to be regripped for the first lesson. I wore my leather glove to pull the trolley from the clubhouse to the driving range, knowing I wouldn't require either the glove or any of the borrowed clubs.

For the first 15 minutes I insisted on the importance of basic warm-up exercises based mainly on what I had seen on Sky Sports the night before. It was during the last rotation I 'tweaked' my shoulder, complaining of a historic, repetitive, and frustrating pinched nerve. Although disappointed, she was sympathetic and understood why I shouldn't demonstrate any further but only observe and 'tweak'.

My chin was raw by the end of the lesson. I must have told her 60 times to keep her head down. All 60 times, she had kept her head down. But she felt there had definitely been an improvement in her game, tipped me £10, and astonishingly, booked me in for the same time the following week, wishing my shoulder a speedy recovery and the prospect of a round soon.

As the weeks passed, my private tuition client base steadily grew until I was out on the driving range teaching more than the pro was. The more I taught, the more rounds I was invited to, and the more elaborate my excuses became. It got to a point where I couldn't remember what I had said to which member, so I ended up having multiple fictional shoulder injuries, all running concurrently and all at different stages of rehabilitation. I used to make myself scarce when I saw three of my students having a drink at the bar together, fearful that I would get roped in to answer some very uncomfortable questions.

Two months in and I had yet to play a round with the pro. The third time I cancelled, he was not best pleased. He had made it perfectly clear that he and I should play a round before the upcoming annual pro-am tournament, where we would tee off first as the rest of the club watched on in awe through their recording phones.

As the day drew ever nearer, ideas on extracting myself with dignity whirled around my mind. Standing on the first tee in battered trainers, in front of my clients and the entire club, hacking away at a driving range ball with my grandfather's bamboo putter was not an option. By now, my feigned shoulder injury had begun to wear thin and foxed one member specifically. She was a physiotherapist by profession and had repeatedly offered a discounted rate, only for me to politely refuse for one bogus reason or another. She had even offered to look at it during my lunch break, and the more I declined, the more her suspicions grew. It got to the point where whenever she came into the shop, I would creep into the stockroom and peer through the door's small circular window waiting for her to leave before sheepishly reappearing.

The shame and guilt I felt saying goodnight to everyone on the eve of the tournament knowing fully that I wouldn't be standing on the tee first thing in the morning, was almost paralysing. To this day, every time I drive past the golf club entrance, I cringe, remembering the inexcusable embarrassment I must have caused and, no doubt, the damage to so many golfers game.

My grandfather's putter still stands proudly in the corner of the garage but now has a glove perched on top. I've also acquired another driving range ball unearthed while out dog-walking, doubling my collection. Although that wasn't the end of my involvement with the golf club, Lady Luck had other designs.

DO NOT TRY THIS AT HOME

'LOST: Black and white dog, blind in left eye, half right ear missing, no tail, limps. Answers to the name of Lucky.'
– **Newspaper advertisement**

I WOKE WITH a swollen, weeping right eye and despite several soothing eye bathing attempts, it felt more comfortable, tightly closed. So be it; these natural occurrences happen at my stage of life, and I went about my daily ablutions, as usual, thinking a strong coffee would stir it into life.

Later that day, Mum and I were picking up my Australian cousin on a break from her self-discovery tour of Europe at the local train station and then driving a couple of hours to Longleat in Wiltshire, so that she could get grainy footage of wolves for her mother back in Australia. Her train was due to arrive at 10.45 am, and we guaranteed her over-anxious mother that we'd be there in plenty of time to meet her. No problem. No worries. Throw another shrimp on the barbie.

But first, I had Anton to walk.

My latest find was a wide bridleway that snaked away into the green unknown. Both sides had thick, impenetrable hedges and a seemingly inescapable corridor for Anton to bounce off without concern. It was still too early in Anton's cultural rehabilitation for him to realise the dangers of chasing anything that moved, and so to him, everything was on the menu. We weren't too far down the track when Anton struck his familiar hunting pose;

his nose high in the air, ears cocked, not listening to a bloody word being bellowed at him. Off he went, through the slightest hole in the hedge.

Seconds later, panic set in as I heard high-pitched, choppy barking and the clatter of hooves on concrete. Unable to fit through the impossibly small hole or see what was going on, I ran down the hedgerow to find a suitable entry point before something lost its life.

I finally found the barb-wired, locked, six-bar steel gate and, with stressed squeals and shrieks ringing loudly in my ears, attempted to vault the gate. The gross overestimation of my athletic ability saw me catching my crotch on the barbed wire, ripping an eight-inch tear down the inside leg of my trousers.

Hidden from view behind the hedge were goats of all different shapes and sizes. Their pungent aroma was cat-nip to Anton, and as he closed in, I ran to intercept him. This was when I rued my dodgy right eye and truly understood the evolutional brilliance of binocular vision and the necessity of depth perception. I came in too hot, too hard, braked far too late, slipped on the piss-sodden concrete, and ended up sliding on my arse into the fence behind. As the goats scattered and Anton cowered, I sat up and somehow found my head stuck between two electric fences. I'd got a smooth C in G.C.S.E. physics, so I knew that one false move would see my head involuntarily and indefinitely pinged between the two currents. As I sat there as still as I could, I thought that maybe Lady Luck had presented me with an opportunity. Having tried most therapies for depression, one I hadn't tried was Electro-Convulsive Therapy, and what with the N.H.S.'s lengthening waiting lists and budget cuts, here was my ludicrously foolish, amateur chance.

After a calculated risk assessment, I opted against lasting brain damage and carefully untangled myself from the national grid, lassoed Anton, and spent two worrying minutes delicately manoeuvring my ripped, piss-saturated jeans back over the barbed-wired gate.

Arriving home late, frozen and with my right eyelid spelling out the alphabet in Morse code, I was greeted by a massive bunch of roses in the hallway. The accompanying card wished Mum a happy birthday with love from my sister in Australia. Removing my glove, I tenderly took a stem and, placing the semi-open, red flower beneath my nose, inhaled deeply. Instead of being overwhelmed with its fragrance, I felt a sharp scratch. I withdrew the flower to see a small but unmistakable bee dangling from my right nostril. Even before I had detached it, I could feel a growing tingling sensation in my nose. By the time I had driven to a nearby Boots in search of an antihistamine, I resembled Gerald Depardeur. Combined with my swollen eye, the right side of my face suggested a baseball bat had beaten me. On reflection, my distorted nose, swollen right eye, and bloated right cheek was an early preview of what was to come. In truth, it was uncannily prophetic.

The short drive to the train station with mum was quiet and, to be honest, a little hairy. With my right eye now firmly closed, and my bulging nose whistling with every inhalation, it probably wasn't the greatest first impression of the UK family branch, so when we arrived late to collect her, she was not only a worrying shade of blue but very probably wondering what sort of inbreeding went on over here.

The onward leg to Longleat was, well, another quiet one, aside from the howling whirl of the car heaters as they did their best to defrost our antipodean relative on the backseat, who had her eyes fixed on me in the rear-view mirror. After adjustment, I then found her eyes on me in the side mirror, shamelessly wandering over my face with a morbid curiosity, too polite or embarrassed to ask any questions. I didn't help the situation by being too polite and embarrassed to provide any answers, and so the seemingly never-ending journey continued without discussing the elephant man in the car.

Restored back to living colour, my cousin snapped away busily on the back seat, whooping in rapture at anything that moved, oblivious to my problems at the front behind the steering wheel. Not only was my one eye having trouble negotiating my way around stationary, stubborn monkeys who refused to leave the road, but I was also preoccupied with a particularly aggressive splinter group that was hell-bent on writing the car off entirely. Reluctant to pay for a replacement set of wipers, an aerial, both bumpers, and four hubcaps, I gently increased my speed. There was something very satisfying about watching the last two roof offenders slide clumsily down the back window empty-handed and out of sight. Safely out of the wildlife enclosures, we parked up the car and made our way over to the imposing stately home.

I'd never attended an Edwardian-themed Christmas before, and as I wandered around, I was only partially persuaded they had fully committed to it. The rooms looked similar to my previous visits, and nothing seemed any different beyond the odd, festive 20th-century battery-operated flame candle.

It took me, my one eye and wheezing nose until the third room to realise the staff in Edwardian costume qualified it as a themed occasion. I was reticent and self-conscious to make conversation at first, but after cutting my Edwardian teeth on the weather with the 'maid,' strolled more confidently into the next room, feeling my dialogue could be more adventurous. Sure enough, as the next 'maid' continually made and remade the bed, we sparred in our ridiculous, unrealistic Edwardian accents covering a whole manner of fictional subjects, from how many fictional geese they have on the estate to the fictional funeral of her fictional husband who had a fictional job working in the fields with their fictional children. She wouldn't break character despite my rapier wit, inaccurate historical quotes, and period ignorance. Her professionalism only motivated me for the next room.

The next room's set-up, however, was very different from the previous rooms. Instead of finding 'maids' doing menial tasks, the only figure I could make out in the gloom was sitting in a high-backed, gently rocking chair, facing a log-burning fire. Being the only one in the room, I had the stage to myself. Rather than approaching the chair, I stood back, taking my time to really suck in the atmosphere, to feel what she was feeling, what it was like to be wearing what looked like a thin, poorly fitting cotton dress on a freezing winter's night. The following interaction is according to my closest recollection.

'How are thou on this wintry noon milady? Wisely tucked up to the fire, I see.'

I waited.

'I said, milady, how dost the day treat th…'

'Fuck off, you perv.'

I was outraged that she had broken character so abruptly and offensively, and so approached her to express my disappointment. I was going to start with how inauthentic I thought her Nike trainers were, but stopped when I saw the baby clinging to her bare bosom.

'Jesus Christ! Can you fuck off please before I call someone'.

With hindsight, I should have stood my ground and calmly explained the confusion but being fully aware of how grotesque my disproportionately asymmetric face looked, especially by firelight, I decided it would be in the interest of both parties if I creepily withdrew back into the shadows, unseen and out of the room, through the exit into the darkness of the crisp, winter night, via the inevitable, outrageously over-priced gift shop.

Two freezing hours later, my mother and cousin returned to the car imbued and impaired, having consumed numerous mulled wines while strolling around the grounds admiring illuminated, festive inflatables. I kept quiet and drove. As I thawed out, my one eye darted between the lines on the road and the eyes in the side mirror, which had taken on tired, unshakeable gaze, highlighted by the headlights of passing cars. To this day, I think it was an irresponsible, minor miracle we made it home intact, and I have rarely been so happy to turn off my bedside light than I was that night.

A month later, we received a warm letter from my cousin sincerely thanking us for one of the most standout days of her European adventure and how determined she was to return to

Longleat. She also wished me a speedy recovery from whatever I was suffering from.

Since then, I have had a new-found respect for people that wear patches. Pirates, James Bond baddies, and poor old one-eyed Willie, I salute all of them, it can't have been easy, and I can now see why they made those difficult life choices.

DEVON HEAVEN

'No man needs a vacation so much as the person who has just had one.' – **Elbert Hubbard**

HAVING TOLD MYSELF I needed a relaxing break from my 11 am alarm and the trials and tribulations of daily dog walks in God's garden, I booked an overnight stay above a pub in the quintessential fishing village of Lynmouth, Devon, a county close to my heart.

It wasn't an ideal start to the day. Baboo, our rebuilt Frankenstein cat, had for the first time in his six years left a deposit in my washbag overnight, which was, regrettably, only discovered when retrieving my toothbrush. To compound matters, Anton, while out on the morning walk, endeavoured to cover his entire body with a badger turd so enormous you could have skied down, and then embedded the excess into my late grandfather's Mercedes 260E 1989 hay-coloured back seats.

Windows down, sunroof open, mint in mouth, all failed in masking a truly satanic stench. The obligatory traffic jam at Stonehenge and midday sun only contributed to the building nausea. Eventually, we arrived at Lynmouth and immediately made a bee-line for the shoreline in an effort to make Anton less offensive before we booked into our accommodation. As Anton frolicked in and out of the waves and the brisk sea breeze blew upon my face, I could slowly feel myself starting to unwind.

Alas, it wasn't long until my zen moment was rudely interrupted by the one question no dog owner ever wants to hear.

'Who's fucking dog is this?'

I turned to eye a huge man further down the shoreline, waving his arms and ominously wading out to sea in Anton's direction. At first, I couldn't see the problem. Anton was about 30 yards out, swimming serenely, parallel to the shore in miles of open water, causing no problems to anyone whatsoever. What a prick.

With night falling and the bitter cold of the Atlantic biting me through my trainers, I was delighted when he beached 50 yards from me, but then saw the 15-foot, bent fishing rod he was dragging behind him. It was then I began to thoroughly understand, sympathise and even agreed with the angriest man in Devon and a lot of his industrial language; although not enough that I wanted to stand around and discuss it with him. I frantically released Anton from his nylon bonds with my trusty, rusty car key and hurried back to the car. I turned to see the luckless fisherman emerging from the water gesticulating in my direction and then empty his woefully inadequate Wellington boots.

I was thrilled to finally book into our quaint, dog-friendly accommodation, 'The Rising Sun', and having washed away the previous forgettable five hours and fed Anton, we made our way downstairs for the evening meal.

The bar was low and beamed in the authentic Devonshire style, and as it was quiet, I decided to sit at the bar, Anton wrapped contently around my feet. The barman was friendly enough. He asked the usual questions about where I was from, what I did etc., and whether I'd seen the signs currently banning dogs from the beach. I nodded confidently as a responsible dog owner. As he passed me the menu, he apologised for not being able to offer the 'catch of the day'; his usual fisherman had told him that a 'dickhead dog had bent his rod, and the dickhead owner had cut his line.' I shook my head as the irresponsible dog owner.

In light of this new information, I retired Anton to the room, returned, and retreated into a dark corner of the bar, exclusively ordering out-of-character large rum and cokes and a baked camembert for my evening dinner. I knew neither what time I got to bed nor indeed how. My last memory was singing along to Elton John's, 'I'm still standing'.

I was wrong to think the cliff-top walk would clear my head the following morning. An hour in, I found myself breaking out in a cold sweat on a narrow, stony cliff-face footpath, trying not to be distracted by the rocks 200ft below or by the mountain goat I'd inadvertently challenged to a Mexican stand-off in front of me. No good ever happens when there's a goat around. Anton knew it too. He had taken to hiding behind my legs, hoping for invisibility. With the wind whipping around my ears and unable to move forward because of my horned nemesis blocking the path or back because of my non-existent hung-over balance, I decided to hold my ground and wait it out, determined to impose my status as the apex species. Well, as it happens, goats have patience. Goats have A LOT of patience. A fact I was not aware of. When it slowly lowered itself, folding its legs underneath without breaking eye contact, I realised I had a worthy adversary in front of me.

At the point I could no longer feel my extremities, I had to concede that he had bettered me and so, inch-by-inch, clinging the rockface, I arrived back down at sea level frozen to the bone, genuinely thankful to be alive, and in desperate need of anything but a large rum and coke.

Recovering by the pub's log fire, I spotted an advert for massages pinned up on a corkboard. After confirming its legitimacy with the barman, I used the pub phone and booked an appointment later that afternoon.

With Anton back in the safety of the room, I headed off to my massage, conveniently a few doors down from the pub.

The masseuse was a lovely lady in her mid-forties who invited me into her tastefully decorated front room, beautifully equipped with scented candles, some distorted whale music, and an impressive collection of various massage certificates adorning the walls between expensive-looking floor to ceiling curtains.

As I lay face down on her massage table, eyes staring at the floor, I became acutely aware that something within me was awry. The first indicator was when my stomach lurched from one side of my body to the other, followed by a deep, seemingly endless Barry White grumble. The second stomach shift pushed an involuntary pocket of air out, much to my embarrassment but, more worryingly, out of my control. I was soothingly told it was 'rebellious chi' escaping and to relax. The third twinge made me clench my buttocks so hard I thought I would give myself a hernia.

When the second groaning dose of 'rebellious chi' burst out moments later, I knew I was fighting against time, and if I had followed her instructions to relax, she would have been in for a very nasty surprise.

I slid myself off the table at such a speed that I took the towel tucked into my pants with me, and as I hurried, still clenching towards the door, the trailing towel pulled two candles off their stands and onto the floor. While she threw dirty vase water on the candles before they ignited the nearby curtains, I frantically searched the corridor looking for the toilet. Third door lucky, bowels bursting, I had no time to lock the door before the first wave came. As I hadn't knowingly consumed any laxative, it dawned on me that cheese wheels washed down with substantial amounts of rum and coke, an early morning death walk, and a massage are incompatible partners.

I paid the now not-so-lovely lady the full amount for my 10 minute 'massage' and tipped her generously for ruining her toilet and for the pooling candle wax on her carpet. On returning to my accommodation, I spied the looming silhouette of the fisherman from the previous night holding up the bar. Having already survived two near-death experiences that day, I decided not to flirt with fate by having a final drink at the bar, gathered Anton along with my belongings, settled my tab with the receptionist, and crept out the backdoor.

On the bright side, at least I know that if I'm ever constipated in the future, I know precisely how to uncork myself. It might not be the healthiest method, but it's undoubtedly the most effective.

NATURE BITES BACK

'I am at two with nature.' – **Woody Allen**

THE WEATHER WAS glorious, so glorious that long-forgotten sunglasses had to be dusted off to deal with the intrusive glare of the low winter sun. As I set off from the gravelled car park across the freezing fallow fields, ghostly white wisps of the thawing earth spiralled ethereally heavenward, evaporating in the cloudless, azure sky. With joyous birdsong as my soundtrack and Anton by my side, I couldn't have wished to be anywhere else.

My chosen path meandered gently through a frosted field before being met by a rusty, tetanus-inducing kissing gate, at which point the trail takes the traveller on a short but steep ascent to the summit. On conquering the lung-bursting climb, survivors are rewarded with a majestic 19th-century stone bench to catch their breath while taking in a spectacular, panoramic view of the Surrey hills.

As I was sitting, heart-thumping, enjoying the vista, a small bird caught my eye. To my delight, the bird turned out to be none other than the British favourite, the robin, enhancing my already contented state of mind. I curiously watched as it hopped around, pecking in vain at the unforgiving ground, occasionally pausing to tilt its head suspiciously at any sudden movement. Sitting statuesque, eyes alert but gladly hidden behind darkened lens, I could hardly contain myself as the robin inched his way closer.

I'd seen documentaries about robins befriending people, and thinking that the stars must have aligned for me to experience a life-changing, spiritual moment, I carefully raised my right hand from my knee, slowly extending my index finger to make an impromptu perch for my brazen feathered friend. Two yards away and edging closer, his tiny, swivelling head suggested he had clocked my digit of friendship and was momentarily considering his options. Three determined hops later, he was on the arm of the cold stone seat and one hop away from me reaching nirvana. Willing him on, I attempted to communicate through a pursed-lipped, high-pitched whistle which piqued his interest and left us beady eye to human eye for a second or two. As he ruffled his feathers, I readied myself for his landing. Wings fluttered. It was happening. Wings fluttered again. It was definitely happening. I felt the air move past my right hand, then right ear. I glanced upward to see which alternative perch he had decided upon, only to be welcomed with a twitch of the tail and an unleashing of the bowels. What came out of that robin was proportionally and physically impossible to comprehend and, certainly not spiritual. If the theory that a bird shitting on you brings luck is sound, I could expect nothing but good fortune for the next five lifetimes. My sunglasses looked like they had been dropped in a tin of white emulsion. When I found myself bursting a robin-effluent-nose-bubble, I knew any chance of enlightenment had passed me by. In celebration of his sudden, dramatic weight loss, the robin erupted into melodic song, happy as Larry, then disappeared into the bushes, not to be seen again; the little empty shitbag.

My mood had somewhat dipped after my avian assault, and the failed attempts to wipe myself clean with a non-porous acrylic sleeve only worsened my spirit and left me with a pagan, war-paint design. To limit possible contact with anyone, I stayed off the main path, making my clumsy way down through layers of dead leaves and sleeping woodland, uncontrollably gathering momentum until I was spat out onto a path right in front of a terrified Hunter wellington and wax hat-wearing, middle-aged woman and her cowering, chocolate cock-a-poo. The scream was, no doubt, justified. If a sweaty, hooded man dressed in black with a smeared, whited face almost fell on top of me in a creepy wood, miles from anyone and anywhere, a scream wouldn't be the only thing escaping from me. Anton was close behind, which at least went some way in alleviating the notion that I wasn't a shit–painted wild man of the woods who laid in ambush for lone females to walk past. I spluttered my apologies for startling her, which were, to a degree, dubiously accepted. In the meantime, her cock-a-poo was straining at the lead, frantically searching for an assumed misplaced tennis ball.

Having already made her reach for her phone once, I tried to make amends and began hunting for the rogue ball. Anton's mincing walk gave away his pride at having found something, so I set about chasing and shouting at him that it wasn't his, and it belonged to the lady as she stood, watching on bewildered. Eventually, after a flurry of obscenities and extended apologies, I grabbed him by the collar and led him over to the woman and her obedient hound, sitting patiently by her heel. To my surprise, I reached into his mouth and extracted the ball with scant resistance. Alarm bells should have rung. As I held it in my gloved hand, I could feel the texture, temperature, and tension was not that of a regular tennis ball. So, with both of us staring on as if I was about to reveal the world's largest diamond, I opened my hand, not to a manky tennis ball but a freshly fashioned ball of horse dung.

The once welcome, awe-inspiring sunlight highlighted just how recently it had been prepared as pillars of gaseous, organic matter clouded the space between her and I. Her 180° spin was so ferocious and sudden she very nearly decapitated her poor dog on the end of the lead.

I returned home, glad the walk was over, and wondered what else the day would throw up. On opening the front door, I heard raucous laughter and the dulcet tones of the Bee Gees seeping from the lounge like a treacle sponge. I slowly opened the door and poked my head in to find my mother and a friend wobbling around in the middle of the room, both with a large glass of rose in hand. Oblivious to my presence, I watched my mother's friend blurt out,

'Ina (my mother), do you know you have a prawn on your shoulder?'

There on her left shoulder was a raw king prawn affectionately hugging her like a long-lost lover. Not knowing where to begin, I quietly closed the door behind me unseen, and went to put my muddy walking boots in the garage, where for weeks, we had been trying to humanely catch the culprit that had ploughed through an entire 20kg bag of dried dog food within a couple of days. Boots down, I went to inspect the trap. Expecting to find a rat the size of a mongoose, I was thoroughly underwhelmed to discover a very relaxed average brown house mouse looking back at me and didn't see the need for the deer's hide gloves that were on standby. That was a mistake. No sooner had I picked up the trap and opened it for a closer inspection, the mouse saw its great escape moment but, instead of making its way to easy freedom, decided to attach itself to the end of my index finger. Instinctively, I shook my hand and sent the mouse to orbital. Out of sight, Baboo had been watching it all unfold from under a superfluous dining room chair and came at my head like a rabid, flying fox, breaking his leap by digging his claws into my scalp. There followed an almighty Tom and Jerry tussle in my hood ending with the mouse evacuating both bladder and bowel as it escaped down my bare back and into the garden with Baboo in hot fruitless pursuit.

As I stood showering, I marvelled at my ability to achieve yet another personal milestone. In just over an hour, I had metaphorically or otherwise been shat on by three different species.

DOGS AND DICKS...

'Some people get so rich they lose all respect for humanity.'
– Rita Rudner

IN MY ENDLESS quest to find meaningful employment, my next roll of the dice bucked the trend of shitty jobs. Whilst out walking, my sister bumped into the force of nature that is Willow. She ran a successful dog-walking business, and although I had seen her out walking, I knew Willow from my bookshop days. She had been a regular customer with eclectic tastes who, with her larger-than-life personality always made her visits memorable.

After a brief informal drink at a local pub with her and her other walkers, Tim and Jenny, I was offered a part-time role, sharing the van with Jenny 3 days a week. The prospect of wandering for hours through the Surrey countryside, through field and glen, with dogs as company, away from any madding crowds, and getting paid for it, was my absolute dream profession.

Initially, I was to shadow Tim, getting to know the regular dogs, their owners, and the necessary admin before his move to London. The dogs came in all shapes and sizes, much like the owners and their bank accounts. From the outset, it was clear that the wealthier the client, the harder it was to be paid. Two dogs we walked daily belonged to an estate that included a moat, an outdoor swimming pool, an indoor swimming pool, a tennis court, a five-a-side grass football pitch, a sunken trampoline, a dozen bee-hives, and a nine-hole, par three golf course. There was, of course, the walled vegetable and herb garden and the apple orchards where a couple of peacocks would often be seen leisurely roaming; all the while, an army of specialist contractors floated about, keeping it all in tip-top condition.

The young lady of the house spent her time sitting on her magnificent Macbook Pro in the kitchen, head in hands, agonising over her creative writing course, having total disregard for the strangers wandering in and around her house, busily assembling fresh flowers or restocking the already bursting, temperature-controlled wine cellar.

When the monthly invoices were sent out, she'd go predictably quiet. Months of texting, emailing, phone calls, and even face-to-face reminders would be answered with heartfelt apologies and broken promises of immediate payment until her debt had grown so large, we had to contact her stock-broker husband, who would issue further embarrassed apologies on her behalf, but more importantly, would pay. She punished us by suspending our service for a couple of weeks, and then the cycle would start again. At the other end of the humility scale was a single elderly lady, working two jobs. Without fail, she left cash on the kitchen table, a loving note wishing good health and a happy walk, and on occasion, a bottle of wine or tin of Scottish short-cake as a gesture of her gratitude.

After the best part of a month, it was time for Tim to leave for London, so in appreciation for his service and a smooth transition, our little dog-walking troupe was invited to Willow's house in the middle of nowhere for drinks and buffoonery.

Tim picked me up, and we made the drive in high spirits. We hadn't been there long when there was a thunderous knock at the back door. Willow excused herself and pulled the door behind her. As Jenny, Tim, and I made merry, we heard an explosive row break out in the kitchen. An angry Liverpudlian accent was demanding to know,

'What the fuck was going on?'

He had seen two blokes arrive and, as her boyfriend, he had a right to know what she was up to. Her chilling, wall-wobbling response somewhat killed the party mood.

'What the fuck are you doing with that axe?'

It was the first time I had been out socially in weeks.

'Where are they? In there?'

Willow, in all her hippy, wholesome wonderfulness, is loving of all things living, plant and beast alike, and aside from the variety of flora she nurtures and grows, inside and out, she regularly adopts injured and orphaned wild creatures, rehabilitating and releasing them back into their natural habitats. Her latest patient was 'Franco,' a young, grey squirrel she had been nursing back to health for six weeks. She had found him abandoned and dangerously weak, but having been treated to an all-day, protein-rich nut buffet, he had turned into the hulk of grey squirrels that stalked people from on top of the kitchen cupboards. You would hear a scrabble of tiny feet from somewhere above and then a glimpse of grey in your peripherals, leaving you feeling exposed and vulnerable. During his recovery, he had also grown fiercely possessive of Willow, frequently flinging himself at anything and anyone that posed a threat to his male dominance, including his own mirror image.

All of a sudden, the drama in the kitchen took a different, equally foreboding turn, and fearing he was on an axing rampage, Jenny leapt from the sofa and opened the door to a lilliputian bald man, psychotically flailing a small axe around his pin head, screaming in a somewhat higher pitch than he had been conducting his earlier argument, for someone to "get it off". Thin scratch marks on his wrinkled forehead were starting to leak red. 'Franco,' having made his successful assault, had returned to his kingdom above the kitchen cupboards and sat on his hind legs, tail twitching, licking his front paws, looking very pleased with himself for reducing this axe-wielding, hard-man manic to tears. After nearly Van Goghing himself several times, he was gently persuaded to relinquish the axe and was escorted out of the door, flapping his arms around his head in a paranoid mess. Once the locks on all the doors and windows had been triple-checked,

Willow's primary concern, apart from her boyfriend being a lunatic, was how on earth he had managed to get to hers so rapidly after Tim and I had arrived, considering he only had a push bike and lived in a town 35 miles away. The night never really got going after that, so when it was time for me and Tim to say our goodbyes, we left Willow issuing assurances that it hadn't been a typical evening.

Willow's concerns about how he made the ride over in miraculous record time were well-founded. A couple of days later, she found a filthy sleeping bag and pillow under her bedroom window. She never saw him again after that night; no doubt too shit scared of being attacked from above to return. As for 'Franco,' he eventually outgrew his empire on top of the kitchen cupboards and left in search of other souls to save. He didn't go far though, as she often still sees him around her garden, watching over her, and each time she does, she nods and thanks him for averting a probable bloodbath.

...DICKS AND DOGS

DOG WALKING IN the Surrey hills has both advantages and disadvantages. Being a designated area of outstanding natural beauty, it is indeed beautiful with forests and heathland aplenty. But it's also a highly populated area, and regardless of how hard one tries to escape others, there's always someone around the corner.

Having been caught short and unwittingly exposing myself numerous times to surprised families, I found myself going further and further off-piste in my search for solitude. However, each and every time, no matter how remote, I'd always cross paths with someone. On one walk, deep in the middle of some ancient, unspoilt woods miles from anywhere, I bumped into a well-dressed elderly couple with their two black Labradors. As the man began going into too much detail about their daily constitutional in perfect BBC English, he was interrupted by his wife bursting into laughter, saying,

'Doesn't that remind you of our first gangbang, darling?'

Behind me, all seven dogs in height order, were vigorously mounting one another. They were all at it, from 'Dylan,' the labradoodle at the front, to 'Matty,' the jack russell at the back. It was as if they were on stage auditioning for Britain's Got Carnal Talent. It was an unforgettable scene, as was the unsavoury image of the elderly couple partaking in their 'first' gangbang.

It wasn't only sexually adventurous old people popping up in obscure places. On three separate occasions, I've been eyeball to eyeball with startled deer escaping pursuing hounds. One cornered so quickly, it was unable to adjust its line in time and leapt over me so closely I could clearly distinguish that it was a healthy, adult male in rutting season.

There were also other surprises, namely wealthy people on horseback. Foolishly, I had begun to listen to music on my walks, so I didn't hear the freakishly large, white stallion approach me unseen from behind, and it was only when I saw Anton hurtle off through the undergrowth, tail between his legs that I turned around. My reactionary squeal made the beast rear up, hooves flailing, forcing its Napoleon in drag, female rider to cling on for dear life. Once she was back on all fours, she suggested in the very plainest of terms that I should remove my head from my bottom and be more courteous to other countryside users. I stood there and took it, more concerned about my peaking heart rate and the state of my underwear to engage in irrational conversation.

After she had blown herself out, the horse and its ragdoll passenger were off, through the wood, over a five-bar gate, across a field, and gone. I continued the walk with my nerves shot and my earphones tucked away in my pocket, anxiously peering over my shoulder every few metres. Nearing the end, and with the sanctuary of the van in sight, I caught another glimpse of the stallion in the distance, trotting elegantly towards an array of outbuildings in the corner of an unassuming, barbed-wired hemmed, grassy meadow. While thinking what enormous stables, I heard the distinct rumble of a plane's propeller firing up. Out rolled a two-seater, yellow bi-plane that taxied its way to one end of the field, accelerated down a roughly cut strip, and disappeared through a gap in the trees at the far end of the field, probably to France to do some duty-free shopping and a lengthy liquid lunch. There aren't any police in the sky after all.

The home of the he/she rider/pilot and the world's most expensive shop is the small, sleepy, linear village of Hambledon. It's littered with 10-digit coded gates that open to Feng-Shui designed driveways that lead to million-pound properties and perfectly manicured gardens. Such are the size of some dwellings and grounds, you would be forgiven for thinking that residents probably weren't aware they had neighbours, let alone answer their rallying call on a freezing mid-winter's day.

After a ridiculously chaotic and brief interview with a new client, I took charge of a small mongrel, 'Trevor,' an American rescue that had recently arrived in the village with his American owners. Usually, a meeting of due diligence is arranged before any new client's dog is walked, but on that occasion and only that occasion, that crucial introduction was bypassed on the grounds of mayhem. Removal men, tilers, a kitchen designer, carpet fitters, and the owner holding a screaming baby on each hip, loudly directing operations from the top of the stairs made introductions less than ideal. With a combination of treats and gentle coaxing, it took nearly 20 minutes to entice 'Trevor' to join the others in the back of the van. Getting him out however, was considerably more straightforward. In fact, it took him less than 2 seconds to rapidly exit the van and less than 5 to completely disappear from view in the abundant undergrowth.

I wasn't expecting much of a response when I asked a friend to post an SOS on the community Facebook page two hours later. Oh, ye of little faith Ben, how wrong I was. The speed and size of the turnout was staggering. Outside the military, it must have been the quickest mobilisation of civilians in peacetime. Villagers regarded it as a call to arms, their duty to be part of the search and rescue; several took time off work to join the operation, and like worms coming out of the ground on a rainy spring morning, there were Range Rovers, Labradors, and cravats suddenly everywhere. A key characteristic of 'Trevor' that the owner had failed to mention was 'Trevor' would only respond to *his* call and *his* call alone and would never approach a stranger; leaving people creeping around in silence with torches on their heads late into the freezing evening.

The following morning, they were back in greater numbers until eventually, 3 miles away and 36 hours after fleeing the van, 'Trevor' was cornered by a driver, cold and exhausted but otherwise fine. And, as suddenly as they had appeared, the village disappeared to await their next community emergency.

As a gesture of goodwill, I charitably decided not to invoice the owners for 'Trevor's' 36-hour walk, suggesting we should probably part ways. While losing a dog on a walk is bad, I kept reminding myself it's not as bad as gaining one. Although the ordeal had been personally stressful, it had, in retrospect, also been one of the most selfless and inspiring displays of human collective empathy and concern for an animal they didn't know, that belonged to a newly arrived villager they didn't know, that I'd seen in a long time.

YOU MAKE ME SICK

'A widespread taste for pornography means that nature is alerting us to some threat of extinction' – **JG Ballard**

As MUCH AS I loved working only three days a week, I found myself cash poor and time rich and so began researching writing avenues to supplement my dog-walking income. It didn't take long to establish from the kindle bestseller lists that the world has an insatiable appetite for erotica. All kinds of weird and not-so-wonderful erotica. Some authors make a tidy living writing about the strangest things, but then again, it's all about suppling the demand. Everything from being tied up by horny werewolves to an octo-dicked octopus has been written, bought, and fantasised about. It truly is a bizarre world out there, and then I contributed to it.

I chose to target a more 'traditional, conservative' heterosexual audience. I was averse to just writing 'porn' for men, that idea made me feel seedy and queasy, so I tried to convince myself if it was written from a *woman's* perspective, it wouldn't be 'porn' but tenuously blurring the lines of 'art.' The most successful downloads that I had read, for market research purposes only, I hasten to add, had all been written by authors with exotic stripper names and mostly from a woman's perspective. Already feeling dirty and ashamed, I sat down to create 'art.'

I spent considerably longer twiddling my thumbs (that's not a euphemism) thinking of my sexy nom de plume than I did outlining the filthy, ridiculous plot. My confidence as a woman had been severely rocked by my last disastrous outing as 'Yoshiko,' the beautiful Japanese geisha, so getting back in touch with my femininity proved harder than before.

Without any knowledge of women's fantasies, I set it out to be a concise short story, but as I started tapping, the plot thickened, and words came remarkably easily. I would even go so far as saying that I was enjoying the experience until having to go into graphic sexual detail from a woman's point of view, not once but many times and in so many different ways.

The intention had always been to write a one-off short story for a 99p kindle download, but as the characters and plot continued to develop, I decided to make my lewd tale into a trilogy. By the end, I was so revolted with what I'd written I could only stomach doing one edit before I hurriedly published them, and as far as I was concerned, that was it. I couldn't even bring myself to look at the sales figures. Honestly speaking, I'd found the whole process rather traumatic and concluded that there must be a better way to make a living that doesn't make me so nauseous.

A month or so later, I was having a drink in my local when Richard, a happily-married friend, asked whether I had any writing in the pipeline. Being a couple of pints down, I foolishly told him about my brief foray into the world of adult literature and, as he's been a faithful fan of my writing, disclosed the series title and excused myself for a toilet break. On my return, I found Richard, where I'd left him at the bar, on his phone. I tried twice to interrupt him, but to no avail, so patiently waited for him to finish whatever urgent business he was so deeply engrossed with.

He put his phone down and stared at me over the top of his glasses.

'When's the next one due out?'

My stomach dropped.

Out of other's earshot, I frantically tried to impress upon him that he wasn't in my targeted demographic, and it was purely a writing exercise. If I thought he would download them, I would never have given him the name.

'Yeah, I understand,' he says, looking at me intently.

'So, when's it out then?'

I spent the rest of the evening convincing him it was simply a writing exercise. In fear of word spreading, I made a grovelling plea to him to keep the title and my pseudo-name confidential which he agreed, on one condition: he would be the first to know if and when future instalments would be published. Thus far, we've both honoured the arrangement.

Richard is and will be the first and last person who knows the name and title. I never discuss it with friends or family, and not even my mother knows I receive a higher monthly income from that 'art' than I do from all my other writing combined. My point is, there are a lot of randy people out there, so the next time you find yourself on a train, sitting next to someone reading a kindle, keep in mind they might just be having the best part or three best parts of their day.

AIR BNBALLS UP

'No amount of time can ever erase the memory of a pet cat you loved, and no amount of masking tape can ever remove its fur from your couch.' – **Leo Dworken**

DETERMINED TO LENGTHEN Anton's life by escaping the neighbourhood's November 5th celebrations, I booked an overnight Air BNB glamping experience back down in the depths of deepest, darkest Devon.

Unwilling to revisit the pastures of clandestine hormonal mistakes, I headed to an unknown postcode that the sat-nav refused to acknowledge. Unperturbed by modern technology's shortcomings, I printed out the ever-reliable AA router planner: no batteries required, just paper, ink, and a sense of adventure. Plans were drawn up to head off the following morning, but before then, I agreed to make up numbers playing 5-a-side football that evening for the first time in 23 years with friends 20 years my junior. A decision that I was to regret.

With the morning sun streaming through my curtains, my head was awash with grandiose ideas of how brilliant our brief, best-friend bonding expedition would surely be. As I swung my legs out of bed, all excitement evaporated. The stiffness and soreness made me check that I hadn't had a double leg transplant overnight, and the usual 6-seconds it takes to get to the bathroom became a gruelling 4-minute SAS training ordeal. If I thought the 7 meters to the bathroom was tough, nothing could prepare me for the stairs. After several futile attempts at descending the traditionally orthodox method, I opted to pull myself down the stairs on my stomach, bypassing any leg usage but incurring savage carpet burns to both nipples.

Two hours late, my hound, my useless pins, and I were on the road, until the first garage we came across. Having filled the Mercedes enormous petrol tank, I very slowly made my way across the forecourt to pay. A lady who must have been pushing 85, leaning heavily on two walking sticks with advanced scoliosis smiled and, without sarcasm, quietly asked whether I needed to borrow them as I was clearly struggling more than she was. I had managed only a few more yards when she passed me again with the distinctive demeanour of someone who had seriously mistimed their toilet run.

I loved my grandfather's car, it was an heirloom, but being 30 years old, she had her quirks. One of her peculiarities just so happened to be unreliable starting, and today was one of her off days. As I sat in the garage's forecourt, desperately hoping for the engine to turn over, a battered white van pulled up to the pump beside me. Seeing that I was going nowhere, the driver jumped out, disappeared around the back of his van and remerged holding jump leads. Gratefully, dutifully, and without a word being spoken, I popped the bonnet. No sooner had the leads been connected, he was confronted by an irate garage employee. It then became evident that neither spoke English as a first or common language. The employee's animated gesticulations strongly indicated he had taken exception to the sparks that had fountained off the engine and onto the forecourt floor, feet away from one of the sixteen pumps.

I sank lower in my seat, pumping the accelerator pedal harder.

As arms whirled and tensions rose, another weathered bloke climbed out of the van, sending the apoplectic garage employee berserk. The second chap was happily chatting away on a mobile phone in one hand and mindlessly playing with a burning cigarette between his fingers in the other. Meanwhile, my right calf had to cramp.

Before anyone was incinerated, my mighty German beast

growled into life. By then, the argument had progressed to involve all three men, all enthusiastically trying to make their point at the same time. When the driver detached the leads and slammed the bonnet, he was so preoccupied with making himself heard, he missed my hand of gratitude as I inconspicuously rolled out of the garage. I watched in my mirror as both parties 'wished' each other a good evening with a flurry of internationally known hand gestures and went their separate ways.

Finally, the open road…

…well, until Fleet services an hour down road that is, where I had to empty my little girl's bladder. Driving around the car park, spaces were sparse, apart from blue-badge holders who had the pick of the place. With my bladder screaming at me and my legs feeling like brittle spaghetti, I had no choice but to park bang outside the stairs to the entrance, in the best blue badge disabled space.

The agonising trip to the gents consisted of lurching from one wall to the next, dragging my redundant legs behind and breaking into a sweat you would rarely see outside a Swedish sauna. Having had a mostly successful visit, I stumbled back to the car, looking like I was wearing callipers under my jeans. On arriving at the top of the stairs, I saw the loathed lone figure of a traffic warden stalking slowly around the car, peering in the windows suspiciously. Pleading for him to wait, I latched onto the aluminium handrail and mostly slid down the stairs towards him. Seeing my sopping tee shirt, my radish-red head on the brink of bursting, and the sheer enormity of effort, he not only stopped writing out the ticket but kindly helped me down the final two.

With the threat of an outrageous fine at stake, I neither confirmed nor denied any diagnosis or the seriousness of my disability, but my genuine inability to walk unaided seemed to satisfy him that I was indeed a more than worthy blue-badge holder, and as he hadn't yet confirmed the ticket, he cancelled it. I thanked him as if he had given me a winning lottery ticket and avowed that the application for the blue badge was top of my priority list. I left the services financially intact but morally bankrupt.

By the time we left the A38, the dark had descended, deeming my AA route planner plan somewhat flawed. The car's interior light had diminished years earlier leaving me in pitch darkness. My decision not to bring my phone had started to smart.

My plan B was as equally incompetent.

With just the village name to go on, I reasoned my best course of action was to drive along the endless Devonian lanes, stopping and inspecting each and every signpost by the flame of a match in the blind hope my village miraculously popped up. With my sense of adventure seriously waning, the sight of dim, multi-coloured string lights of a village pub was most welcome. The gravel car park was auspiciously empty, and the pub's tired, wooden façade was slowly being taken over by swathes of thriving green moss. Inside, faded beer mats covered low black beams, and the heavily stained, worn, 1980s-patterned red carpet was peppered with missed crisp fragments and historic cigarette burns. The black and white photographs of pretty girls sitting on workmen's knees which covered the walls suggested the pub's heydays had long been and gone.

Sitting on a stool at the end of the untended, dimly-lit panel bar was the pub's only patron. He was an elderly man in his 70s or 80s wearing a tweed flat cap, a thick white beard, and a stare that hadn't left me since I'd walked in. While he watched my every move, my eye caught what he had at his feet, rendering me momentarily motionless and forever perplexed. It was a cat but not your average moggy. This cat was stationary mid-stride, its mouth permanently ajar and its tail stiff as a hairy aerial.

'Takes it everywhere with him' said the portly barman, who had appeared from the cellar, smiling.

'Has done for years, haven't you little Pete?'

Little Pete's scrutiny of me continued.

'He don't talk much to strangers. Says he'll never need another cat.'

As I approached the bar, I saw that the cat's feet had been

crudely nailed to a board of splintering plywood. The thinning hair and bald patches on its back and underbelly paid testament to decades of love and hundreds of miles of affectionate carriage. I remember standing at the bar, staring down at the cat, trying to evaluate whether I loved or loathed the idea. Little Pete had a pretty solid argument after all. I had completely forgotten why I was there when the barman asked whether I was there to eat.

As it happened, Lady Luck had been on my side. Remarkably, I was only a couple of villages away from where I needed to be, and as the barman reeled off directions, I could feel my gaze returning to the stuffed cat.

Having thanked the barman and wished little Pete and his cat all the best, I sat behind the wheel of my car in the quiet darkness of the desolate car park for a couple of minutes, waiting for my brain to process one of the strangest pubs I've ever seen, reviling myself again for not bringing my mobile. I had always thought nothing would beat the dead, two-headed, five-legged goat I'd seen in a Burmese market, but I had been wrong. I had so many questions. Had it even been his cat or had he bought it, found it or inherited it? How old was it? All questions that still keep me awake at night and I'll never know the answers to. I continued on through the lanes in the vague direction the barman had pointed, distracted by the cat's snarly expression which I couldn't get out of my mind.

The final 500 metres saw Anton and I travelling over rough, farmland, dodging sheep and rabbit holes like I was playing an arcade game. I was beginning to think I had been led up the proverbial garden path when the car's headlights fell on our final destination; a lowly, basic, humble shepherd's hut. Located on the summit of a windswept, barren hill, the disintegrating, rusted orange corrugated roof served only a slight purpose, as did the rotting, antiquated wooden door, flapping on one bent hinge in the blustery, northerly wind.

The 'bedroom with a stunning view' had been a tenuous, economically truthful description at best. The narrow space consisted of a child's 5ft Disney 'Frozen' mattress, covered in a cracked, protective plastic, which in turn was covered by an entire ecosystem. The 'stunning view' was of the doorless, barely standing, meagre wooden shelter 10 meters opposite that housed a composting toilet and two buckets, one full of sawdust and the other of rank-smelling water. None of it even slightly resembled the provocative photos I'd seen online.

While making the unenviable decision of whether to sleep with Elsa in the devil's armpit or spoon Anton on the backseat, the first firework was heard.

Anton did a 'Trevor' and was gone.

Two hours and several painful laps of the field later, after my fingers had turned blue and I hadn't felt my face or feet for hours, I found him curled up, fast asleep on Elsa. I decided against catching worms with Anton and spent the remainder of the night sitting bolt upright in the car's passenger seat, wrapped in a moth-eaten removals rug that had been in the boot since the early 90's, freezing my carpet-burnt tits off, dreaming of little Pete's cat.

The next morning, after having left what I thought of the stay in the toilet, our next priority was to find the day's first food. Even under an iron sky, escaping the high-rise hedges and rivers of unmarked tarmac took an eternity, pushing breakfast into brunch and then lunch before we found a food-serving pub.

The one mini cherry tomato that made up half of my £6.95 cheese and tomato sandwich neither satisfied my hunger or my idea of value for money and was the final straw that broke my tired, stiff back. First, the undeserving waitress and then the manager received both exhausted, hungry barrels, ending in a full refund and the promise never to return.

Twenty minutes later, I re-entered the pub, convinced I'd left my wallet on the table. When it wasn't, I struggled my way over to the stony-faced barman, sceptical that someone hadn't picked it up in the brief time I'd been gone. He regarded me carefully then asked the waitress to tend the bar as he reluctantly came over to help with the search. My almost complete immobility saw him crawling around under the tables on his hands and knees, when in a pocket I could have sworn I'd checked, I fondled my wallet. My attempts at apologetic small talk and congratulations on a wonderful customer service were met with an equally stony silence as yet another furious stranger gave me a warm, two-fingered send-off.

Once more, Lady Luck unequivocally demonstrated that any visit to Devon is always richly rewarded with lasting, death-bed memories. Since I have returned to the parish of Wormley, I can't tell you the hours I've spent pouring over regional maps and satellite imagery, vainly trying to find that pub again. It's as if the village, the pub, little Pete and his stuffed cat had disappeared into the ether, into the mists of one of Devon's many Bermuda triangles. Something tells me I could spend the rest of my days driving around those lanes searching for little Pete and his stuffed cat and never set eyes on them again.

LUXURY IN THE HEART OF THE FOREST

'I hate people. People make me pro-nuclear'. – **Margaret Smith**

WITH MY SISTER, niece and nephew coming over from Australia to stay for a couple of weeks, Mum went into overdrive organising indelible family days out. Time with them is so precious that she would move sun and moon for more of it and spends hours researching suitable venues, looking for that perfect experience. In the recent past, we've been truly fortunate to enjoy family holidays in some, quiet, breath-taking locations, so it was quite a surprise to both my sisters and me when she asked us to clear our diary for a trip to the gem in the crown of domestic staycations; Centre Parcs.

She had booked 7 of us into a woodland lodge for three days and three nights at the Woburn Forest site in Bedfordshire. On hearing the news, my Australian sister's response, 'I can't think of anything worse,' seemed somewhat pessimistic at the time.

The first indication that maybe mum had missed the mark was the traffic queue that snaked miles from the entrance. With it being the height of summer, some cars hadn't fared so well in the blistering heat and sat on the roadside, engines steaming while their sun-glassed, topless occupants lay on the grass happily turning tones of crimson. Many appeared perfectly content to be seated on foldable chairs, car radio blaring, tearing into giant bags of Wotsits, as their young children chased each other with water pistols.

When both cars had eventually made it through the imposing entrance gates, which made checkpoint Charlie in Berlin look like the gent's turnstile at Waterloo Station, throngs of partially clad bodies bobbed along in a slow, relentless march. Most were on foot, but some cycled around on hired bikes. Convoys of wheeled families weaved their way through the crowds, mercilessly cutting other families in half, separating mothers from the handles of their prams and fathers from their sense of humour. In the time it took us to find our lodge, I must have heard 50 small children screaming at fallen ice creams and adult language that's banned on the stands of the most hostile football matches.

Having checked into our woodland lodgings, we re-joined the masses in search of our reserved bikes. Such was the acreage it didn't take long to realise we needed a bike to find our bikes. Every few yards, colour-coded signposts pointed down other congested avenues, which had further crammed paths sprouting off them and disappearing over the humming human horizon. We knew we had found the bike rental simply by the size of the queue. The couple in front of us had planned ahead with a complete picnic hamper which they casually kicked along, regularly reaching in to retrieve chilled Scotch eggs, homemade cheese and pickle sandwiches and cans of alcohol-free beer.

The skinny teenager and only employee at the bike stand, had been all but consumed by the overwhelming volume of inquiries and had all lost control of which bikes were coming in and those going out. Bikes on bikes, people on bikes and people on people surrounded him as he spun around with a clipboard, absorbing frustrations and apologising on behalf of the company.

With a set of wheels, next on our agenda was a dip in the communal pool. Having consulted the indispensable map, we arrived at yet another queue for wristbands to gain entry to the changing room and its miles of numberless lockers. As I wandered around the maze of locked lockers, looking for a vacant one whilst dodging wet children duelling with foam noodles, the unease of what awaited beyond the changing room doors grew. Fearing for my towel's security in the great unknown, I locked it safely away with the rest of my belongings in a locker before taking a deep breath and heading through the swing doors to the pool area.

I was greeted by nightmarish bedlam. Sleazy strangers, lone rangers, children with parents and grandparents, young and old couples of all shapes and sizes covered almost every inch of everywhere. I've seen cobwebs that offer more coverage than some of the swimming costumes, and others which would be illegal in 95% of the world's communities. I stopped outside the doors to compose myself, and nearly lost my toes to a mini spiderman who had commandeered a mobility scooter and was forcing everyone in his path to take drastic evasive manoeuvres. One small girl, wearing union-jack armbands and holding hands with her grandparents were all sent for an involuntary dip in the mums and babes pool as the scooter and its rider veered off into a wall. The two pursuing security guards first waded their way through the slippery, wriggling bodies to help the stricken trio to their feet before confiscating the scooter and threatening the potty-mouthed superhero with a banning.

There were, of course, more queues. Queues to the slides, queues to the toilets, and queues to join other queues. The wave pool looked like something out of North Korea, with rows upon rows of bodies bobbing up and down, all facing the front wall in eager anticipation of the wave machine starting up again. Now and then, people passing would detour into the pool, shuffle in up to their belly button, stand statically, staring into the middle distance and then climb back out, negating any need to join the ever-growing toilet queue.

Overhead, different coloured waterslides twisted and turned, spewing sliders out at such regularity and speed it was difficult to establish where one body ended and the next began. It was like a never-ending human centipede. Waterslides have never been my thing. They've always worried me from a young age, when I was told by some bastard that people deliberately stuck chewing gum on slides and then stuck razor blades in the chewing gum. I'm sure it's an urban myth, but it's still there in the back of my mind, waiting to prove that prick right one day. The only queue I was big-boy brave enough to join was a slide that took the swimmer outside but, more importantly, had a restricted age limit, so no babies on breasts or terrorising, little Jonny shitbags; an adult's only slide if you will and by the time I was shot out at the bottom, I could see why. After a gentle beginning, it gradually quickened and narrowed, funnelling the unsuspecting slider into several dangerous bottlenecks along the way. Swimmers would gather and writhe like salmon in a holding pen while waiting for their turn to be popped out into the next stretch whilst all the while being battered by the constant stream of people coming behind. Nearing the end, a rough, concrete section of the slide cornered at such tight angles it became more about self-preservation than thrill-seeking enjoyment. Aside from negotiating a potentially concussive blow from the wall, I was ever mindful of the flailing stranger's feet, a yard behind my head at any given time, and travelling. When I was ejected out into the bottom pool, it felt like the 20-stone, hairy bloke wearing the world's smallest trunks had hit terminal velocity when his heel struck me on the back of my head.

I'd had enough fun when I saw two grave-faced employees carrying first-aid cases, weaving their way through a concerned crowd to one of the slides exit pools and hurried off to the changing room, nursing two grazed elbows and a throbbing head. While I couldn't get out of there quick enough, Lady Luck had other ideas. As I wandered around looking for my lost locker, it dawned on me that I was no longer in possession of my wristband. I'd only been on one slide once and it had taken me a whole 15 minutes to lose it. I mentally retracked, wondering whether I'd lost it on the death-slide or been robbed by the Spiderman scrote on the scooter.

Reception was…to be expected, heaving, with no one staffing the front desk. Being the only half-naked, dripping person there, I could feel every part of me shrinking with each passing minute as my shivering took on such vibration, it looked like I had early onset of Parkinson's. Forty minutes later, after answering some tricky security questions, I was allowed back into the changing room. It then took a further 10 minutes and 200 locker attempts to find mine and my most welcome towel.

As for the rest of the family, well, they enjoyed the water facilities longer than I did, especially my niece and nephew, who, from Western Australia, had never seen so many strangers willingly rubbing up against each other in one place, and found the whole experience a novelty, a novelty which quickly wore off. 4 hours after their return to our lodgings, my niece first complained of stomach cramps. An hour after that, so did my nephew. A further hour later, both hugged the toilet with tears in their eyes. Such was their rapid deterioration; the on-site doctor was cautiously called who told us it was a 'common occurrence when children get together' and had nothing to do with the gallons of piss they had just absorbed. That effectively ended my sister's, niece and nephew's 'holiday' at Centre Parcs and whilst they spent the remainder of their time under duvets, watching movies with a bucket next to them, I had activities booked.

Venturing out, only when absolutely necessary, I made my way to the eagerly anticipated, pre-booked and paid-for 'archery experience.' Loud klaxons should have sounded when, for the first time since I'd been there, I hadn't had to join a queue. In fact, the only queue of note was that of parents, excitedly jostling for position behind their cameras, behind their respective child. I've always been interested in all things middle-ages and from an early, lonely age, made my own bows from chopped yew, arrows from Hazel, flights from foraged feathers and bowstrings from local Devonshire horsehair, hence, I was slightly disappointed when I was handed a pink, rubber bow the length of my forearm, powered by an extra-large, blue elastic band bowstring. Before the 8-year-old boy, two 10-year-old girls and I were given our completely inoffensive, 6-inch, sucker-head rubber arrows, we had to complete a 30-minute safety briefing. The entire 'experience' was only 40 minutes. You would think that I would be exempt having survived to middle-age, but despite my more than reasonable protestations, I was cynically informed, 'everybody has to complete the safety induction before they can use the weapon.' He was the only 'weapon' I could see. Sitting cross-legged on a chipped, stone mushroom a foot off the ground, he went along the line, asking us farcical safety questions. My question was to point at where I thought my eyes were and then I was asked why we shouldn't shoot each other in the eye. He corrected me on my answer.

After graduating third in my safety class, we were given our five arrows and sternly told to wait as he put the targets out. Five yards ahead of me, he placed a six-foot cardboard cut-out Peppa Pig while my fellow archers were given Sponge-Bob SquarePants, Barney and Fireman Sam to target. Only when he was 'safely' behind the line could we load, not fire our bows, until given the order. My first arrow barely made the distance, landing on the hessian matting at Peppa's feet which halted proceedings so that he could give me a not-so-welcome lesson on how to pull back a bow and aim.

I left with a lolly, an attendance certificate signed by Disney's Robin Hood, and a total conviction that 15 years spent fending men off in showers would be totally worth seeing Peppa shoved up his arse.

We left as we had come in, queueing for just as long and feeling a little sorry for the stationary queue going the other way. In the car on the way home, I asked my sister whether she had enjoyed her three days at Centre Parcs and the same sentence she prophesied all those miles away was repeated, 'I can't think of anything worse'. Amen to that, sister. Amen.

WITLEY CRICKET CLUB

'Villagers do not find village cricket funny' – **John Arlott**

THERE'S SOMETHING TRIBAL about twenty-two, mostly hungover men in twenty-two thickly knitted jumpers huddling uncomfortably close to one another, cursing the April weather and quietly questioning local pub opening times.

I'm a member of the mighty Witley cricket club, aka the Witley Weasels, Witley wieners, or Witley #ankers, depending on the game's result. Over the last couple of decades, my youthful ambition and passion for the game had slowly ebbed away and I had been more than content to keep abreast of the game watching it from the comfort of an armchair in the lounge. That all changed walking back from the pub when I literally stumbled into an evening net session and was invited to hurl down a few drunken deliveries. An hour later, having lost a stone in sweat and Anton sporting a red-leather hue around his mouth, I dubiously agreed to play the following Saturday, knowing next to nothing about the greatest cricket club in the world.

Founded in 1869 by a clear visionary, it's the oldest, finest, and only cricket club in Witley, Surrey. Whenever possible, the club fields two teams that play in the *daddy* of all leagues, the I'Anson, which according to its website:

'…believe the league (founded 1901), which draws its member clubs from Surrey, Hampshire and Sussex, to be the oldest continuously-operating village cricket in England, and possibly the

world.'

The league is relatively competitive, and whilst Division 1 enjoys aging, half-senile, impartial, paid ECB umpires, the lower leagues rely on players' unbiased honesty to officiate. Except, there is no honesty in village cricket. Batters regularly smash the cover off the ball to be caught on the boundary, 60 metres away, only for the batter to insist they hadn't touched it. More often than not their team-mate umpire sides with them, regardless of how ridiculous and always to the verbal fury of the fielding side.

No umpire will ever be as memorable as the one who officiated my debut game. Having dug out my dated whites, yellowing canvas pads and broken-handled bat, I was given the ambiguous privilege of opening the bowling. Considering the only leather I'd thrown in nearly two decades had come from a legless arm, it was a perilous move with which I wholeheartedly disagreed. Nevertheless, the new ball was thrust in my hand and as I wandered around guessing at my runup, the umpire brushed past me in his white jacket to place the bails on the stumps. Just as I thought the butterflies in my stomach couldn't get any more rampant, the umpire turned to ask me my bowling action. He hadn't managed to complete the first word when he stopped and stared at me. Of all people, probably in the universe, Lady Luck had me face to face with the golf club steward who had diligently driven me around his beloved course. I wanted the ground to swallow me. He never completed his question and turned back, telling the batter not to worry about being given out that over. He was our home umpire. There followed one of the longest, most expensive, exhausting and humiliating overs I've ever bowled in my 36 years of cricketing. When it was my turn to bat, he gave me run out without facing a ball, completing the appropriate and well-deserved lesson. It transpired that he was a respected, highly-regarded senior club member who had been involved with the club for the past thirty 30 years. Each time I saw him thereafter, the enormous golf club bull-elephant which was present in every awkward conversation, was never mentioned.

Our club emblem is the magnificent copper beech that proudly stands keeping watch over the ground like Father Time. Despite its massive length and impressive girth, the colour of its leaves makes for the worst sight screen conceivable. It still astounds me that in the clubs 150-year history, only 40 players and 17 spectators, including the local vicar, have been injured by an errant cricket ball. Out of the 57 injuries to date, the vicar remains the only casualty to require hospitalisation. Fact truly is stranger than fiction.

Aside from the tree, there are plenty of other hazards of which to be wary, namely the showers. We rent two dank, disturbingly dirty changing rooms and four archaic showers from the parish-owned community hall. The showers' temperature fluctuates so wildly that they've become a genuine health hazard with brave and foolhardy participants finding themselves in a constant in-out, shake-it-all-about dance as they do their best to wet their bits without being scalded. From afar, it's reminiscent of a questionable south-Korean game show. During the winter, the 'Witley and Milford Pumas' use the same facilities with marginal success. Judging by the usual hellish aftermath, it could safely be assumed that some live in the woods and have never been toilet-trained or know where to dispose of soiled toilet paper. It's a place where angels would fear to tread and certainly not for the faint-hearted or those who aren't entirely up to date with their vaccinations. The home changing room regularly features piles of damp, sweaty, neglected clothes that fill the air with a noxious, nauseating, acrid odour. Visitors are advised to wear face-masks until properly acclimatised.

With games being usually played on a Saturday, the rest of the building, including the veranda, is invariably hired by a wedding party. By agreement, when required, we have to request anyone involved in the cricket, including the opposition, the scorers, and spectators to relocate to 'the long grass' in front of our carbuncled, decrepit machine shed until the contest's conclusion.

The machine shed is also our castle. It's the one erection we can call our own and houses all that is precious to the club. It's a run-down, dilapidated, 5m x 5m breeze-block monstrosity of a construction, barely standing, but it's ours. Inside, buckets of cobwebbed cricket stumps sit alongside three broken, 19-century mowers; two absurdly heavy, rusted mystery machines and a diesel-powered tarmac compressor from the 1950s, which is used as our roller. She's also lethal. To start her is taking your life in your hands. Car battery leads are attached to effectively jump-start her, and unless you know what you're doing, there's a very real danger that you could get seriously singed as she blows you against the wall. If you're successful, you have a tiny window from starting her in gear to getting behind the controls. The cracked brickwork on the back wall offers clear evidence that not every driver made it in time.

Our outfield is managed by the parish council, which means every Tom, Dick and Mary is welcomed and encouraged to use it, and everyone and everything does. Foxes, badgers, rabbits, cats and dogs. Lots of dogs. Lots and lots of dogs. Whereas rival teams employ groundskeepers to tend divots and the odd weed, we arm players with buckets and spades to tackle the turds and raze the mole mounds. It is, as we say, 'the Witley Way.'

Along the lower boundary runs an established hedge that claims countless cricket balls every season. At various points during every game, there will be a row of men on their knees blindly fondling the hedge in the hope of a lost ball. Aside from the blackthorn, brambles and barbed wire, lurk other dangers.

A couple of seasons ago, while searching for yet another well-struck ball, I snagged the back of my hand on what I thought was a particularly vicious thorn. Withdrawing my hand, I found two distinct, puncture wounds but as we were in a rare commanding position over our nearest rivals, carried on with the game. By Monday, my hand had ballooned to cartoon proportions and was in urgent need of a medical professional. After a lengthy examination and some confusion, I was given a two-week course of antibiotics to treat a false widow spider bite.

Over the venomous cricket ball graveyard lies a maintained gentry estate where fat sheep lazily graze around a large lake that a pair of pure white, majestic swans call home. On the lakeshore, dozens of plump Canadian geese stand asleep, gracefully balanced on one leg, heads buried deep in their plumage, fearing neither the threat of man nor beast.

On the other side of the ground, the busy Petworth Road runs parallel to the top boundary, separated from the playing surface by a Grade II, 15th century, listed wall. If the wall belonged to Hadrian or the Chinese, I would respectfully understand and let it be, but it's a bothersome wall, high enough that the only people capable of overlooking it are, more often than not, van drivers. Opinionated, vulgar van drivers who, in the space of 90 meters and 6 seconds, let everyone know what they think about cricket or 'croquet' as some simple folk shout. They don't always have the last laugh though, as any sweetly timed shot puts passing motorists directly in the firing line. To date, one motorcyclist, three cars, and a bus have been taken unawares by a travelling cricket ball, one even landing square on the passenger seat through an open window.

Beyond the wall and road of obscenities lies a large meadow gently sweeping from right to left up to a high Scot's pine treeline. During spring and summer months, wildflowers and grasses blanket the earth where crickets and the buzz of wings provide a restoratively soothing soundtrack and in the autumn months foragers and recreational mushroom pickers take great, hallucinogenic delight in filling their punnets and laughing at clouds. On warm, clear, mid-summer nights, the bright, moonlit meadow transforms into a magical secret kingdom of childhood wonderment. Feathered and furred beasts alike roam about their nightly business under huge, star-studded skies. It's one of those very few places where you think if you stayed long enough, you'd see mythical creatures and gnomes holding midnight court.

For cricket, you would also think having a flat or near-flat playing area would be obligatory. Not for the mighty Witley though. Such is the severity of the undulation of our ground, there are certain fielding positions that aren't visible to the batter in their crease. I've witnessed players standing, admiring the shot of their life, waiting for the umpire to raise his arms for six, only to be horrified when a fielder emerges from a misty hollow to claim the catch. There have been heated calls for these hidden ninja fielders to wear a festival-inspired, high-flags to show their fielding whereabouts. Negotiations are ongoing.

The league's photographer is also worthy of note. He's an interesting, well-known character that has been travelling between the grounds for as long as anyone can remember. With his Simon Cowell under-nipple, cord trousers fighting to contain his burgeoning belly, he creeps around the boundary taking action shots for the local paper. He also has an uncanny ability or sixth sense to show up at exactly when tea is taken and often comments on what treats other teams have had on their tea menus, in an effort that we up our game for his next visit the following week. But despite his eccentricities, he loves the game almost as much as his teas. Long may he live; the league wouldn't be the same without him or his unique eccentricities.

But Witley cricket club is a special place, and I'm not the only one who thinks so. Among the loyal members there's Brutus who's playing his 19th consecutive year at barely 30 years of age and Sarah, who for years, selflessly commutes from Aldershot every summer Saturday, rain or shine to facilitate a game for others.

Amid the occasional encouraging clap, the gentle sound of young families playing and picnicking drifts across the ground. One such family belongs to one of our players. He's a fearfully competitive, bordering on being a wrathful individual and while his mother watches over his young son on the boundary, he threatens the umpire with a stabbing to the eye if the next decision doesn't go his way. Of all the hundreds of hours I've spent standing in my whites, all over the world, one of my most endearing moments has not been with bat or ball but watching him losing his shit as his son ran across the pitch pushing his inseparable baby pink, Barbie pram. His poor mother came under a torrent of abuse for first getting the pram out and then letting him escape onto the ground. The tantrum he threw when they eventually caught him must have been heard miles away. His son's scream when he was separated from his pram was almost as loud. The pink pram remained his son's most treasured toy for three, long years. According to his weary alpha-male father, he refused to go anywhere without it; even insisting on taking it to school and onto the stands of Crystal Palace matches as his fanatical father stood bare-chested, waving his shirt around his head.

Like many other league teams, Witley relies exclusively on volunteers. The work that goes on behind the scenes to get two teams out every weekend for four months of the year is nothing short of Herculean. You would think it would be pretty straightforward to organise 22 grown men to be somewhere at a specific time, but in reality, it's more like herding skating kittens. With player's availability constantly in flux throughout the week, the thankless, stressful task of confirming two teams takes on an evolving life of its own, right up until the first ball is bowled at 1 o'clock on a Saturday afternoon. Despite the restless toil, there are still players who confirm their attendance, express their excitement, get arseholed on Friday night and fail to turn up or answer their phones, effectively ruining the weekend for players and families alike who had committed their best hours of the week in the expectation of a game.

The square maintenance and quality of pitches also lie in the hands of club volunteers. Again, while some grounds have the finances to employ year-round specialist ground keepers, we have a volunteer team of about six that tend our pitch diligently. Over her 150-plus year history, the square has endured just under 2,000,000 cricket balls being flung onto her surface, which has rendered her lifeless to say the least, and regardless of the countless hours of laboured love spent sitting on our 1950's tarmac compressor, she's tired. So tired that balls rarely bounce higher than the knee. Opposition players that come out to bat wearing a helmet are openly mocked.

The dogged determination of the volunteers and club members not only to keep their club running but to keep improving and moving forward, inspired me to be a Witley cricket club representative on the Chichester Hall committee in the hope that we'd get a say in the facilities which frequently wounded, and the length of the long grass which we were routinely banished to. Seven of us reluctantly met once a month. I was 30 years younger than the next youngest woman and one of only two men. The other gentleman was an emaciated, suited and booted, silver-haired, beaten husband of an elegantly dressed, busy lady that wore her grey hair up in a tight bun. He came under a constant barrage from her, never more so than after he'd had his fill of tea, biscuits and cakes and sat at the table, dozing and interrupting speakers with a snorting piglet noise. The wife would wake him with a sharp, bony elbow to the ribs, prompting instinctive apologies before he closed his eyes again and slipped back into semi-consciousness. One woman took obvious exception to the treatment of the hen-pecked husband and so took it upon herself in making life as difficult as possible for the wife in the time she had with her. Everything, absolutely everything had to be debated, debunked or disagreed with, from the colour of the hall's toilet paper to the origins of the pencil. The meetings became so long and predictably pointless that one woman used to dip into a book when the conversations erupted. It was a scene straight from 'The Vicar of Dibley.'

Progress was stalactite slow. It took six arduous months to get an approved electrician to change a light bulb. My offer to do it, of course, sparked an animated war of words between the two aging adversaries, which ultimately had to be decided by means of a vote. I lost the vote, leading to another disagreement about which electrician should be called. I resigned from the committee after deciding it would be more productive and pleasurable to stick my balls in a vice than to endure their endless point-scoring feuds. And so, to this day, the length of the grass permits standing only whilst the showers continue to make the uninitiated dance.

But my crowning glory at Witley came in 2018 when I was proudly appointed club captain. Grand plans were drawn up and ranged from installing non-lethal showers to family pram stands, but alas, I would see none of my dreams realised or even partly so. During the third game of the season, I jumped for an innocuous ball being passed around the field and thought Lady Luck had stabbed me in my right calf with her stiletto when I landed. A grade 3 rupture of the calf muscle, the size of a fifty-pence coin saw me side-lined for ten weeks and the captaincy passed to the vice, who held it for a further two years. In its 150 playing history, I hold the unenviable record for the shortest tenure as captain and statistically the worst. Played 2. Lost 2.

BLUNTY, BOOBS AND BASKETBALL

'So where the bloody hell are ya?' – **Australian Tourism campaign**

PERTH, AUSTRALIA IS a long way from the Surrey hills, in every sense, geographically especially. Unless you're prepared to walk and swim, you'll be spending a long time sitting, and no matter how comfortable the airlines claim their seats to be, 24 hours will test the fitness of anyone's buttocks. I've always regarded the epic-crossing as a trial, a rite of passage, a test of patience necessary to visit one of the world's greatest countries.

That said, I wasn't so convinced of the worth 30,000 feet above Uzbekistan as my unconscious Asian gentleman neighbour blew bubbles on my right shoulder, whilst I worried whether I'd wet the seat, having been numb from the nipples down since somewhere over the Pyrenees.

My two-week objective to the far side of the world was a straight-forward mercy mission; give as much love and support as possible to my newly-single, stella sister and her beautiful children in their new chapter of independence.

The online check-in, two days before the flight, went unerringly well. I reserved my favoured window seat, four rows away from the toilets, close to the exit points, but more importantly, at least 30 rows away from any baby amenities and therefore 30 rows less likely to spend time in a foreign prison for baby air-rage. I also took the opportunity to explore the vegetarian page, which I found to be genuinely bamboozling. There wasn't a whiff of the classic macaroni cheese or the humble baked spud on any of the menus, and so, after considerable consternation, I hesitantly opted for 'Hindu vegetarian', as I'd recognised the word poppadum.

It turns out that my earlier concerns about the trouble-free online booking were well-founded. Firstly, the automated booking-in machine at the airport failed to recognise either my passport or my ticket, putting me at the back of a queue, the size I'd last seen and joined when I lost my wristband at Centre-Parcs. The family of six in front of me, with their twelve suitcases, two double prams, and a 1970's retro food blender the mother cradled carefully under her right arm, was an auspicious start. The only ray of sunshine was watching the struggling father play a moving game of giant Jenga with the suitcases on a stubborn, headstrong trolley. Every time the line inched forward, he would burst into a sort of dance. Steering with his knees, one hand would be trying to release the brake on the handle, whilst his other frantically tried to thwart his travelling tower from toppling on his three-year-old toddler. Despite his regular pleas for help, the mother stood by and point blank refused to be parted from her food-blender, clutching it closer as if she held baby Jesus in her arms.

As we neared the front desk, an airline-uniformed, sharply featured chap in his forties appeared from nowhere at the head of the queue, and began checking passports with such gusto you would think he was looking for America's most wanted. Everything about him was busy. The speed at which he fingered through passports, his darting eyes, and quick, short strides. I don't know what it was with my passport but he handled it like a soiled condom, gripping it gingerly between thumb and forefinger at arms-length out in front of him as he marched on ahead. I eventually caught my breath and up with him at a lonely, unlit desk. My less than polite enquiries on why I had been targeted went unanswered as he entered details onto the computer with such mesmerising finger speed it gave me motion sickness.

He broke his silence by informing me I didn't have an Australian visa and therefore couldn't fly. He had a point; I didn't have an Australian visa. I was absolutely sure I could obtain a 3-month tourist visa on landing. He very much disagreed and sat opposite on a swivel stool, legs crossed, patiently waiting for my shameful list of mistruths and inaccuracies to burn out. Once I'd exhausted myself, he handed me back my passport having not only secured me a Visa but had also rearranged my seating so I had an entire row to myself between Hong Kong and Perth, even further away from any potential infant-related incarceration. He handed back my passport and was gone as suddenly as he had appeared, lost in a sea of stationary legs and lingering luggage.

It was on the first leg to Hong Kong that my Hindu vegetarian decision was questioned. My sense of importance at being served first was short-lived. Peeling back the warm aluminium foil, I realised how precious little I knew about the Hindu diet. Apart from a stray, rogue, loitering lentil, I recognized nothing as familiar or even edible. Having thoroughly enjoyed the lentil, I suspiciously rejected the remains of what was in front of me, pushing the tray to one side and covering my grumbling belly with the complimentary blanket as my neighbour repositioned his head on my shoulder.

Hong Kong airport was, at first, nothing like I had read or heard. After separating myself from my disorientated, disgruntled slumbering companion, I disembarked the plane and followed the overhead signs to a dismal, disappointing lounge with rows of cocooned, sleeping-bagged transit travellers. Even the tired, poorly stocked vending machine looked depressed. For the next four hours, I sat playing snake on my ancient Nokia phone, deafened by *another* Asian gentleman who had found comfort on the same right shoulder.

In need of sustenance, I asked several severe-looking officials the whereabouts of any retail outlets. All seemed bored, some even weary by the question as they gestured heavenward until one led me around a corner and pushed the 'up' button by the doors of the biggest lift I'd ever seen, obscured from view by a poorly-positioned pot of bending bamboo.

When those lift doors next opened, I was momentarily blinded. It was like I was walking into Willy Wonka's chocolate factory. Sunglasses should be mandatory. Not that I got to walk around it. No sooner had my eyes adjusted to the illuminations, my flight number was called. There followed a stiff, sweaty walk from one end of the sprawling airport to the other, finally arriving at my boarding gate to be reminded by the cheery airline staff that I had a vegetarian breakfast to look forward to.

Perth airport by comparison, is positively medieval.

Rather than the plush Gucci and Tiffany duty-free stores, the jet-lagged traveller is greeted with more stuffed koalas and boomerangs that you can throw a stick at. By the time 'Doug' at border control had informally quizzed me on the purpose of my visit, I regarded him as a firm friend and probable wedding guest; such is the welcoming, open friendliness of Western Australians.

Outside the airport, away from the burly beards and finely-tuned Utes, the feeling of open space backs the fact that Perth is the most isolated city in the world. Long, wide, beautifully smooth roads stretch out into nondescript desert wastelands, populated only by kangaroos, wild camels, and psychotic men with a penchant for backpackers.

Rockingham, a western suburb with plenty of beaches, wallabies, snakes, spiders and scorpions, is one of the commonwealth's final frontiers. It's also home to a disproportionate number of tradespeople, clearly distinguishable in their thigh-length shorts, steel-capped boots, wraparound sunnies, and a yellow or orange high-vis, florescent top. They're everywhere. In shops, on the beach, in restaurants, on side-lines watching their son play cricket, in the sea throwing about a ball, at wedding parties, and after a while, every time you close your eyes. All men who aren't poised for immediate groundwork are looked upon with a degree of wariness. I soon realised that you're far more likely to see a man running around with a reinforced bucket on his head kicking down walls, than one wearing a three-piece suit.

Entertainment in Rockingham is somewhat limited. The closest I found to a traditional English pub was the 'Nags Head' which was located just off a four-way, four-laned highway crossroads, next to the drive-through off-licence. Essentially it was one long bar partitioned into two by a retractable, wheeled wall. One half was the sports bar, where jumbo TVs aired re-runs of various Australian cricket and rugby union victories to empty tables under dreary lighting. In contrast, the other half of the portioned-room was absolutely chocka with rows of small TVs on the walls which covered every sport, from trap racing to American football, and next to them, more rows of flickering TVs, constantly updating the changing betting odds. With no tables and standing room only, I've never seen so many high-vis tops in one place, all fully committed to emptying their bank accounts as quickly as possible. Whether frantically feeding coins into a bank of 'pokies' or backing random greyhounds in Japan, it had the atmosphere of a busy sweetshop.

Aside from the losing groans, the only other booming voice was that of a topless, black thong-wearing barmaid calling out meat raffle numbers. It was most peculiar watching her shimmy around the packed room, squeezing herself between the totally disinterested high-vis crowd, yelling out winning ticket numbers and holding up bags of chicken giblets. Once she had distributed her various bits of carcass and offal, she grabbed a baseball cap and sunglasses from behind the bar and strutted out into the blazing sunshine and a waiting car, breasts and buns bouncing around in all their natural glory. It was a lot to take in for early Tuesday afternoon, and what had started out as a quiet drink descended into a determined session.

As I wobbled my way around the pub, one of the conversations I literally fell into was with a lovely, butch, mining lesbian. In truth, we had nothing in common, apart from our mutual love for all things James Blunt and so after trying to harmonise, 'You are beautiful' with her, was invited back to hers with the promise of more booze and Blunty singalongs. Before we left, I vaguely remember asking her how far away she lived and whether I needed to visit a cash machine. 'Just down the road' and 'get fucked' were her respective responses which suggested a short walk home in my addled English mind.

I thought our taxi driver remained remarkably composed, considering our constant heckling to change radio stations and to turn the volume up. I was having so much fun that I paid no attention to where we were going or how long it took to get there. We arrived at her house sometime in the early hours, where a plastic glass of white wine was eagerly thrust into my hand. By early dawn, I was hoarse and barely standing. Blunty had been our only soundtrack as we worked our way through five bottles of wine that lay empty, strewn across a pine coffee table which I had shinned a dozen times.

I was woken by the front door slamming. Opening my lazy, hungover eyes, I was somewhat confused to find myself on the spacious wooden inner window sill in the front room, a meter from the memories of the night before. My searing headache wasn't helped by a close-cropped haired, heavily tattooed woman screaming obscenities at the top of her voice a yard away. During her rantings, last night's friend appeared looking like I felt and began trying to pacify her. She had just finished her shift and was tearing into her girlfriend, accusing her of 'returning to her old bi-ways.' While they went hammer and tong at each other over their sexuality, I mumbled my thanks and left by the front door into the early morning blistering sun.

An hour later, with the sun high in the sky, sweat dribbling down my back and my bald head beginning to blister, I had yet to come across any familiar sights or signs or anywhere that could quench my gasping thirst. When the road I was walking along turned into a dusty track, I started to fret. Through the heat haze, I spotted a parked bus about a kilometre away and hurriedly made my way towards it hoping it wasn't a teasing mirage.

I was within a hundred meters when I heard the bus's engine

roar into life and despite my frantic arm-waving, watched it pull off and away into the distance, leaving me at a remote bus stop, out of breath and out of ideas.

Sometime later, another bus approached and after hearing my plight, the mirthful driver enjoyed explaining that I had walked an hour in precisely the wrong direction and, as he wasn't going that way, helpfully advised I returned the way I came. By now, my exposed torso and legs had taken on an unhealthy, scarlet tinge, but on the plus side, I had at least managed to save my bald head from lasting damage by draping my tee shirt over my head like a blasphemous Mary Magdalene.

Off I stumbled back the way I had come until I was once again outside the house where I had spent the night. As I stopped to collect myself, the angry lesbian just so happened to come out and seeing me, stood and glared.

'What the fuck are you still doing sniffing around here?' she abruptly asked.

'I'm trying to get back to Rockingham. Do you know which way? I…'

'…It's that way…' she sneered, giving me the middle finger.

'…Up ya fucking arse. Dickhead.'

With that, she got in her car, slammed the door and drove off.

Three hours later, I was back at my sister's, dangerously dehydrated, with severely sunburnt legs, arms, back, chest and face. As I recovered, lying head to foot in thick aloe vera, I realised that 'just down the road' in Australia takes on a very different meaning than 'just down the road' in England. The next time I head off into the outback, drunk with a complete stranger, for impromptu Blunty karaoke, it's probably wise to take a phone with a map on it and an SOS option.

Sadly, that wasn't my only drunken escapade while in Western Australia. The other came when my sister and I set off on a quest of reconnection to the world-renowned Margaret River for a wine-tasting weekend. On the way, there were several stop-offs at various small family-run vineyards where grandmothers listened to radios and sold bottles to the public in giant vineyard warehouse shops. As my sister was driving, it was left up to me to do the bulk of the tasting. One particular tasting stands out not for the wine but for the award-winning winemaker himself. He was a brawny, bearded man with slack regard for his appearance, wearing sun-bleached thigh length shorts and a buttonless, open shirt. With some relish, he explained to us that he 'can't stand the stuff' and feels far more at home with a cold can of VB in his hand. It's an unorthodox yet effective marketing strategy that clearly works as our intrigue saw us driving away from his remote warehouse with a dozen bottles rattling around in the back of the car.

I know it's never a good idea to mix drinks, especially in the Australian sun, without eating and not knowing the whereabouts of your accommodation, but sometimes these things happen. My sister had sensibly decided to head back to our lodgings early, leaving me in a Margaret River bar with simple directions scrawled on the back of my hand on how to get back. After time had been called, I stumbled onto the town's only commercial street, forgetting everything my sister had told me. Two words remained legible in biro on my hand, 'Red door'. Two hours later, I was back at the bar where I had started, scratching my head and eyeing up a wooden bench as a bed for the night. But before I admitted defeat, I thought I'd give it one last go, so off I set on the same circular route, inspecting doors more closely as I went. However, my new interest in the local's front doors during the early hours of the morning had attracted some unwanted attention.

To begin with, I pretended I hadn't noticed the police car slowly following me and did my best to hide behind a recently planted sapling that was no thicker than my scrawny leg. When they addressed me as 'the pissed bloke hiding behind the tree,' I couldn't be absolutely sure it was directed at me as I was still well hidden from view.

'Mate, we can see you'.

I waited a moment, hoping someone else would appear from the shadows.

'Yeah, you, the pissed bloke hiding behind the tree.'

I clumsily stumbled out with my arms high in the air, fearing the worst. True to the Western Australian culture, they were the two most amicable, uniformed men I have had the pleasure of meeting. They found my inability to walk or recount anything but a red door highly amusing and kindly offered to escort me as I wobbled my way through town. With dawn fast approaching, I spotted it, concealed by my sister's car, not 50 metres from the bar I had left hours earlier. I thanked my new friends for their protection and apologised for being a tit before collapsing face down on my bed.

After that followed, three blissful days. Hours of meaningful conversation fuelled by mobile baristas, the odd beach walk and wine-tasting, and a sense of timelessness went a long way to re-establishing the deep bond of yesteryear. They remain three of my fondest days.

Like many Australian children his age, my nephew is a keen sportsman. His preferred sport currently is basketball which is hugely popular in Australia. Every weekend, hordes of children and their parents from the surrounding area descend on the local leisure centre to play other regional teams. During my visit, I was fortunate to be invited to one of his games which just so happened to be against a rival team. Teams are kitted out in sponsored gear, have background staff analysing players, teams and trends, a physio, and I even spotted one team with a 7-foot rooster mascot that danced every time its team scored. What I thought would be an easy-going, enjoyable afternoon listening to children's laughter was anything but. On either touchline, friends and family screamed abuse at the referee, the opposition's family and even the players. The officials spent most of their time not officiating but crowd-controlling. It was a gladiatorial bear pit and akin to being at a Manchester City/Manchester United football derby. My nephew's eight years old.

On the court, the longer the game went on, the more physical the game became. What started off as a basketball match, became indistinguishable from of a brutal game of British bulldog by the time the final whistle was blown. But to my surprise, it wasn't the parents' passions that spilled over; it was the coaches. The head coach of my nephew's beaten team charged over and squared up to his opposite number accusing him and his team of underhand tactics and dangerous play. He had compelling evidence. Two of his players had been substituted with bloody noses, another had a bitemark on his forearm and the smallest, a swollen eye that had all the hallmarks of a gouging. The other coach threw a counter-accusation back, leading to the two of them bumping chests like two amateur Sumo's going at each other. After five or ten seconds of this bizarre peacocking, parents united to force them apart and with one more barrage of expletives, they left by different exits, followed by proud parents holding bruised and battered 8-year-old hands.

When it was time to leave my sister and Rockingham, I wasn't sure whether I had achieved my original objective of support; in truth, she supported me while I was there, not only financially but spiritually, emotionally and psychologically. I often rerun the conversations we had while we were away in Margaret River, and each time, I learn something new, something profound, something to marvel at her intellectual brilliance. Saying goodbye to the three of them at the airport was difficult, regardless of the lifelong memories made. I hope to go back one day, and if I do, I'll make sure I'll pack a phone with a GPS and stock up on a variety of high-vis tops.

YOU CAN'T BE SERIOUS

'Unseen in the background, fate was quietly slipping the lead in the boxing glove'. – **P.G Wodehouse**

WE ALL GET headaches from time to time. One particular headache however, never left. I thought the constant dull ache that had engulfed the entire right side of my face was nothing more than residual, unreleased flight pressure in my sinuses or an accidentally inhaled second lentil from my vegetarian meal. Inconvenient but not debilitating, life continued with daily dog walks and daydreaming dawdling's.

When my eye started to involuntarily and, at times, inappropriately wink at people when I smiled, I ruled out aviation air pressure or lentils and reluctantly made an appointment with my G.P., citing probable sinusitis. She disagreed with my unqualified speculation and immediately referred me to the ophthalmology department at the Royal Surrey hospital.

On 11/11/19, I wrote in my notes, '*Unknown facial condition – struggling with severe headaches and facial swelling. Have been referred to the Royal Surrey and am awaiting scans. Loss of appetite and insomnia'.*

Thankfully, I hadn't required a hospital for a while so when I turned up for my first ophthalmology appointment on November 18th, 2019, I was blown away at the insanely busy Costa coffee neighbouring an even busier Marks and Spencer's, where dressing gowns, pyjamas and slippers are not only the norm but expected and even encouraged. In terms of diagnosis, the appointment was disappointing and the diagnosis inconclusive.

On December 2nd, I attended my second ophthalmology appointment. Once again, eye examinations were carried out and passed, and so an urgent MRI was requested with emphasis on the head and the eye orbits. Meanwhile, the swelling on my cheekbone had visibly grown and was now becoming painful. A seven-day anti-biotic course was prescribed.

December 10th: I had my first MRI. It was also the first time I had worn a hospital gown. Do hospital gowns come in different sizes? I tried three and regardless of how I wrapped myself, I always seemed to leave my arse exposed. Paranoid about my dignity, I slid onto the MRI stretcher only to be politely asked to return to the changing room and slip on some underwear, jeans and socks. My embarrassment was soul-destroying.

Once the table had been thoroughly disinfected, the room was cleared of personnel and the MRI machine whirled into action. While the machine does its thing, the patient is in constant touch with the control room through chunky headphones and a small, angled mirror positioned above the patient's head. Every couple of minutes, instructions are relayed as each scan is taken. Midway through these scans there was a pause. As I watched in the mirror, I saw the operator pointing at the screen. Her colleague's words of comfort through the headphones did little to soothe as more and more people entered the control room. At its height, I counted seven white coats crowded around the screen. That made me slightly nervous, which was only amplified when one of the control room staff wished me 'the best of luck' in the sincerest manner.

Two days later, on December 12th, I received a phone call from the radiography department asking me to attend a full-body MRI scan. Considering I hadn't had the results of the first MRI head scan, the request for a full body scan, costing the NHS around £500 at an already stretched hospital, did not bode well. So, 48 hours later, I was fighting with more ill-fitting gowns in a dressing room.

After being discharged from the ophthalmology department, my next hospital appointment was with the Ear, Nose and Throat department on December 16th. I remember sitting in the ENT outpatient waiting room watching people with severe facial disfigurements come and go, thinking I must be in the wrong place or someone along the way had made a mistake. As far as I was concerned, I had an infection and just hadn't found the appropriate antibiotics. For the first and not the last time, I felt like a fraud. I felt imposter syndrome. My swollen cheek didn't belong amongst these people's horrific injuries.

My name was called and I was led to a side treatment room where I was introduced to a young medical student finishing her training and then to a head and neck oncology surgeon.

My heart lurched.

Seeing any surgeon is always slightly unsettling, but a surgeon who specialises in cancer, for me, was a whole new level. He was a relatively young man with a kind, cherubic face and a reassuring demeanour. Before I could digest and query his profession, he swivelled around in his chair to face me.

'So, Mr. Dobson, what have they told you?'

'Nobody's told me anything.'

He slowly turned his screen to me.

'I'm sorry, it's shit.'

He then proceeded to point out a large, dense white mass on the right side of my face stretching from the bottom of my right eye socket, down the side of my nose, along my upper jaw and to my ear. The comparison with the left side of my face was unmistakable and unforgettable.

He drew up his chair, put his hands on my knees, and looked me in the eye.

'As I said, it's shit.'

There was silence.

I had always imagined that when people are diagnosed with cancer, they break down uncontrollably. I felt quite relaxed. At peace. There was a calm, suspended serenity about the moment which I would gladly relive.

The trainee plucked a tissue from the desk and dabbed the

corners of her eyes. She took the news worse than I did.

'Are you sure it's not chronic sinusitis?'

There was another silence.

'I'm sorry, Mr. Dobson. We can't see it anywhere else if it's any consolation.'

'That is good news.' I remember cheerfully saying, trying to disperse the heavy atmosphere.

The remainder of the appointment was a blur. On leaving the treatment room, he emphasised the need to act on this promptly and that I would be sent a letter outlining the biopsy and treatment details. With one more apology and the best wishes from the solemn-faced young doctor, I was on my own. It was a strange sensation. I joined the crowds of people in the miles of busy corridors and drifted aimlessly, in a meditative, emotionless state, without a place to be and without a time to be there. When I did, by chance, happen upon the outside, I bumbled around the car park for 20 minutes looking for the car, only to realise I was in the wrong car park altogether.

The drive home took longer than it should have after I overshot my exit by 30 miles and ended up sitting in rush hour traffic in the next county of Hampshire. I was still in a warm, cosy, calm, timeless, numb bubble and thoroughly content. That time between the treatment room and pulling into the drive at home has been one of the most peaceful windows of my life. Ironically, it was the state of mind I'd been searching for all my life. I'd never felt more at peace than when I was faced with the prospect of death.

Reality returned abruptly as I pulled the into the drive at home. I sat with the key in the ignition, staring at myself in the rear-view mirror, weighing up whether I could possibly get away without telling my mother inside. Such news can be hard on loved ones. The decision was made for me as soon as I opened the lounge door and saw her sitting cross-legged on the sofa doing a crossword puzzle.

'How did you get on?' she enquired, head down.

The tears were already rolling.

'Not great…I've got cancer.' I blurted.

Turning to look up at me through her glasses, her next remark took me aback.

'At least you haven't any hair to lose.'

What else do you say in that situation? It was like throwing a flower into the middle of a fight. It was as baffling as it was brilliant, pausing the tears as my brain calibrated her comforting words. When they began tumbling again, and the incoherent mumbling and uncontrollable shakes started, I was given an early glimpse of my future as an elderly man, which made me cry harder.

One of the hardest things to hear was her wishing she had it instead of me. Of course, it's a beautiful demonstration of unconditional love, but as a depressive, I could think of no better person to have it than myself. It's 'what I deserve.' Much rather me than a happily married father of three.

Mum then had the unenviable task of contacting immediate family with the news. Within the hour, Charmian was by my side and Emma in Australia, at vast expense, had booked the first flight over, essentially and indefinitely putting her life on hold. Their swift, selfless responses reminded me of just how lucky I really was.

On the 19th of December, I was admitted to the surgical short-stay unit for my biopsy and what should have been a stressful time was lightly relieved by a couple from across the pond. With only one unoccupied chair left in the waiting room, I found myself facing a large lady in her mid-50s. Worn, failing shoes exposed her dry, cracked, beefy heels and her weather-bleached blue tee-shirt which she had grossly outgrown, possibly in her teens, doubled up as a makeshift bra. The tight, light linen trousers left nothing for the imagination.

However, what took my eye was not her questionable wardrobe or that she was oozing out across three chairs but rather her seemingly rapid touch-typing technique. In the hour that we sat facing each other, I didn't see her look down at her computer once and yet the speed at which her fingers moved, she could have written the bible twice over. At one point, she expertly opened a Cadbury's dairy milk slab, a tear and share bag of salt and vinegar crisps and sprung a can of coke without her left bunch of sausages pausing.

Her husband, of similar age, was positively skeletal in comparison and poised delicately on the edge of her third seat, one bony buttock on, one bony buttock off, nervously adjusting his stars and stripes braces that did little in holding up his ankle swinging brown cords. His bitten nails and facial tick suggested a problematic marriage.

One by one, we were led to our cubicles. There were six in all, and by lucky chance I was opposite our American friends again. A short-stay unit is pretty much the same as the rest of the hospital wards, with a bed, one visitor's chair, an emergency cord, a table on wheels, and a flimsy, blue paper curtain that runs around the perimeter of the bed, giving to some, it seems, an artificial sense of privacy.

Curtain drawn, it started up again. Tap, tap, tap…

Soon after came their conversation that could have been heard in the middle of a tropical typhoon.

(With a deep southern twang)

'Looks better, ain't it?'

'I ain't no doctor, for the sake of Jesus, son of God, you put that away.'

(Still the tap, tap, tapping continues…)

'It don't hurt so much either...'

'Now, you put that away right now, or I'm gonna slap it away.'

'I's just saying…'

'Well, I's just sayin'...'

All that was missing was a banjo and an unhealthy sexual lusting for family members.

I was the last to go under the knife that day. I came around in the recovery room and was wheeled back to my temporary bay and to the familiar sound of relentless, furious fingers.

Still off my tits on whatever the funky, hot Japanese anaesthetist had given me, I couldn't help but smile wider at the following conversation that drifted upon the airwaves.

'That ain't right; look, is that swelling supposed to be there?'

'Give me strength, Lord Almighty! If you don't put that thing away, I'll give you something that really hurts; now you put it away right now. What would your mama say? God rest her soul.' Every now and then, nurses popped in and popped out with wry smiles on their faces. Judging by their repetitive, sympathising tone, he wasn't entirely happy about what they told him and was eager to get others' opinions on it, including the poor, unsuspecting cleaner who left his mop in the corner to go and find a medical professional.

When it was time for them to leave, the blue curtain was drawn back to reveal him sitting in the visitor's chair and her lying on the bed with the computer and a can of sugar-free Sprite precariously wobbling on her keg of a stomach. As I watched her shuffle to the edge of the bed, she momentarily paused her express typing and rested the computer on the bed long enough for me to see a completely shattered screen, as if someone had discharged both barrels of a shotgun into it. There was no way it could have been working. The white earphones that hadn't left her ears once dangled limply by her side, unemployed, without a listening device in sight. She left the unit being pushed out in a wheelchair, computer on her lap, fingers tapping, earphone port in her crotch, with the poor husband following obediently, albeit gingerly like cactus Pete, cradling what was left of his battered manhood with both hands. Soon after, I was discharged with stitches inside my nose and a very rare smile.

December the 23rd and the pain in my face was increasing at an alarming rate. Paracetamol wasn't cutting it; it was barely touching the sides. I looked forward to my hospital appointment the following day if only to be prescribed adequate pain relief.

Early on Christmas Eve morning, we received a phone call cancelling our appointment later that afternoon. Although we'd avoided spending a large proportion of Christmas Eve sitting on our arses in traffic, I was by then being driven to distraction by the pain that had not only engulfed my face but my entire head. It was a chronic, dull, thudding pain throughout that I can only describe as a hangover headache combined with being repeatedly punched in the face with an anvil. My distress sent mum on a telephone goose chase trying to find somebody, anybody who could help. Eventually, her perseverance paid off when the doctor who had originally diagnosed me, sent through a prescription for Pregabalin to treat the neuropathic pain and the foreboding anxiety. Over the course of the afternoon and evening, both slowly waned until it was bearable, uncomfortable but bearable.

On the second of January 2020, I returned to the Royal Surrey with my sister and mother accompanying me to hear the biopsy results. The surgeon who had performed the biopsy told us that the tumour had been a "highly vascular angry one", and in all his medical years, he'd never encountered one that'd "bitten back." The unexpected 20-minute tussle he had with an uncontrollable bleed that had, at one point, "been of concern."

Because of its unusual, aggressive behaviour, tissue had been sent around the country to form some collective idea of the type of cancer, whether anyone had seen anything like it before and how to go about treating it. The results were expected on the 09/01/20. He did however give the probable treatment plan. Initially, it was likely that chemotherapy would be used in conjunction with radiotherapy to shrink it pre-surgery. As he delicately put it, "we don't want to leave you with a divot in your face" which made me think, I bet there are some at my local golf club who wouldn't mind leaving me a divot in my face. Anyway, until the pathology results were in, he was unable to give a timetable or any details of the treatment plan aside from the chemotherapy/radiotherapy starting in a week or two. It was a thoughtful journey home.

I can't be sure whether it was delayed, ongoing shock or the uncertain future ahead but for a few days my head became… blurred, confused. I ran on a sort of auto-pilot, managing the routine activities but struggling with anything that required one iota of brainpower. One straightforward trip to the shed ended in my mother having to cut me free from the washing line with a pair of secateurs as I didn't have the mental capability to extricate myself.

The 9th came and went without pathology results or a reason for its delay. I still wasn't sure whether I was dying and if I was, how long did I have.

On the 20th, I wrote in my notes, '*People keep telling me to do whatever I've wanted. Must make a bucket list. QUICKLY*'. The problem was, I've never known what I've wanted to do. I *think* I've always wanted to do the Tea Horse Road through Asia and go to Bhutan, but with £2.37 in my savings account and 0.56p in my current account, that seemed a bit of a stretch. With or without a list to work through, my only realistic option with that sort of bursting bank account was half an ale at the nearest Wetherspoons.

On 23rd January, I was given the news that whatever was growing out of my face was beyond the limits of the Royal Surrey and so my case had been referred to the Royal Marsden in Chelsea, a specialist cancer hospital. The tumour by now had grown to the size of large, squashed tangerine.

My inaugural appointment at the Royal Marsden was on 6th February. By road, there and back is a half-day operation travelling through several of London's busiest boroughs. By rail, two hours, and by far the best option if you don't mind your nose being buried in several stranger's armpits for the entirety of the commute, but expensive when travelling with company.

Although I'd previously lived in London for two years, I was unaware that Chelsea has a cancer corner. Cancer research centres, cancer charities, cancer hospitals, and even parking spaces reserved for cancer patients. Despite being surrounded by all things depressingly cancer, the chic French restaurant 'le Colombier' does a booming business. Every time I passed it, I used to look in at the well-heeled clients tucking into fillets of finest beef as taxis and private ambulances pulled up outside to drop off morbidly ill people. Young and old struggling to mount the curb in their wheelchairs, pressing oxygen masks to their faces and pushing their IV drip next to them didn't seem to affect customer's appetites.

My clinic appointment in the radiotherapy department yielded no biopsy results and the pathology results remained unclear. Specialists couldn't identify the tumour, how aggressive it was, or how it would behave during and after any treatment.

They needed a second biopsy to be done.

Now that I was a patient at the Royal Marsden, new bloods had to be taken and tests run, one of them being an ECG, and so after my disappointing clinic appointment, I retook a seat in the waiting room. My name was called and I trotted off to a small room where a camp male nurse was waiting to welcome me. There followed the most awkward 5 minutes I've spent in the company of another man.

Sitting on a black stool, I removed my top as instructed as he fiddled with the dials on the radio. Satisfied with KISS FM, he wheeled himself over holding a yellow plastic Bic razor and shaving gel, triggering memories of the rusty shave I had in a Laos barber's where I walked out with a bloody head and very nearly the owner's daughter as my bride. He hummed away in his own world as he squeezed the gel into his gloved hands, warning me,

'I'm sorry, it might be a little chilly at first…but then some people like that'.

Whilst I stared at the ceiling, not daring to make eye contact, he liberally applied to the gel to my chest. His flamboyant shaving strokes were not those of a nurse but rather those of an accomplished artist. On completion of each pass of the blade, he sat back, tilting his head from side to side as if painting a renaissance masterpiece. Each nipple was dehaired in one fluid circular motion, clearly demonstrating my chest hadn't been his first rodeo. I thanked and complimented him on his professionalism and returned to the waiting room. When I was called the second time to have the actual ECG, the male nurse smiled when I removed my top and said, 'I see that Raphael prepared you'.

On the 11/02/20, I was back to undergo another body MRI and a CT head scan. The day hadn't begun well. Anton's bowels had loosened during the night, sparking a military-style clean-up throughout the house and a complete loss of appetite.

My morning continued in the same vein. Well, actually, that's not true. If it were, the beleaguered yet smiley nurse would have found mine rather than stab in vain at my arm a dozen times to get a cannula in for an imaging dye, all the while telling me to settle back and relax. With her job crudely done, she escorted me to the door and told me to pop along to my MRI appointment. This was the first time I'd had an MRI scan at the Royal Marsden and in my appointment letter, I had been instructed to attend the mobile MRI scanner. Being the dickhead I am, I had forgotten the vital piece of paper with the directions and the map to the mobile unit.

The Royal Marsden, Chelsea, is a sprawling medical metropolis. Across roads, over and underground, through tunnels, and in temporary, semi-temporary and permanent portacabins. It's the chaos theory of buildings. With the cannula hanging out of my arm and no idea where I should be, I asked a beautifully made-up, well-spoken and well-dressed, middle-aged receptionist for her help.

Judging by how the day had panned out already, I was gratefully surprised when she eagerly left her post from behind the front hospital desk and enthusiastically marched on ahead, telling me over her shoulder it was her first day and this was as much as an adventure for her as it was for me. Having weaved and circled our way around several disused and barren outbuildings, my guide eventually conceded and politely interrupted a surprised porter halfway through his Tesco meal deal lunch for directions on my behalf. His vague, irritated finger-pointing seemed adequate for the receptionist to smile and toddle off, overjoyed that she could be of service.

Against the day's grain, I struck gold at the first portacabin I called in until the receptionist asked me to don yet another hospital gown. This particular gown had frayed tassels where the strings were once attached, so when I emerged from my cubicle, my left hand worked to keep the wind from whipping at my inner thigh. The MRI receptionist chuckled and then apologised for the gown's malfunction, but before she could direct me to the scanner, the phone rang, leaving me to find my own way again.

As none of the portacabins were labelled, I tentatively wandered around in the freezing February rain, peering through darkened windows and trying locked doors. When I could see my shaved nipples through my saturated gown, I thought it probably best if I sought assistance and headed for the only door in the only brick building, immediately finding myself face to face with a large man holding a sizeable, serrated knife. I was angrily shooed out of the hospital's kitchen by the same porter who had given me the somewhat ambiguous directions earlier and led back to the portacabin I had just left. After another unsuccessful change of minuscule gown, I was led by the hand of the sympathetic receptionist to another portacabin, where I was asked to change into another less revealing, more hygienic gown before finally completing both scans.

Two days later, on St Valentine's, I was back for a busy, and in no way romantic day. My 2nd biopsy pre-op was at 2 o'clock when I had to answer a belittling questionnaire on my poor lifestyle choices. The self-righteous nurse had already re-educated me on the dangers of my historic smoking and then reprimanded me for the rest of my appalling score. As a lasting gift, she handed me a bottle of 'Octenisan,' a decontamination washing lotion used in preparation for surgery which, once applied that evening, reminded me of the Deep-Heat seniors used to put in my pants at school.

At 2.30 pm, whilst waiting for my appointment, I was approached by a 'Biobank researcher' who diligently took me through all the small print of donating tissue samples to be used for future research and scientific purposes. Her morbid enthusiasm was a stark reminder of just how rare the cancer was.

I met the doctor who was overseeing my care at 3 pm, who

introduced me to the French surgeon that would be cutting up through my upper right jaw to extract another sample for pathology. He was an arrogant prick with an uncanny resemblance to Martin Kove from Karate Kid with zero bedside manner. His staunch insistence that all questions should be referred to anyone but himself didn't help cross-channel relations. Once he had deflected everything he possibly could, he slammed the door behind him so hard that it made the shelves rattle.

My day at the Marsden was rounded off with an x-ray of my teeth, jaw and gums. The radiotherapist took no pleasure in outlining the devasting side-effects radiotherapy can have on components in the mouth, including losing teeth, sore throat, and sore tongue to such an extent a gastro-pipe is inserted to bypass the patient having to swallow. It was an exhausting day one way or another and a harrowing, sleepless night.

Four days later, I was slipping on sexy stockings again for my second biopsy. Considering the complications of the first biopsy, the French surgeon seemed pretty relaxed that a massive bleed would never happen on his watch.

Surprisingly, I woke up. Not only did I survive his butchery but I didn't need a blood transfusion either.

At home, the following morning, the entire right side of my face was three times the size and had me looking like the familiar elephant man who had taken the trip to Longleat all those months ago. My eye was partially closed, my nose was on a kink and my cheek was stretched like a tight balloon. I had expected some swelling but nothing like this. It was so shocking several phone calls and photographs were hastily made and sent to a variety of people at the hospital, enquiring whether everything had gone according to plan when I was in surgery, was the severe swelling normal, and could there be any possibility he had accidentally left a boule or partial baguette in there?

The loyal surgeon's secretary explained that due to the rarity of the cancer, there was no way of predicting how the tumour would react but there were no recorded incidents in the operating theatre and Ibuprofen was suggested for the swelling. I was given strict instruction that if it got worse or too painful, do not, on any account, go to A and E, as it would be too complex for them to handle and I should go directly to the Royal Marsden's pain team.

On 24/02/20, at 11 o'clock, I was scheduled to have my mask fitted. For the radiotherapy's accuracy, a bespoke mask is made, placed over the head and shoulders, and secured to the radiotherapy table by ten robust bolts preventing even the slightest of anxious twitchy-head movements. The fitting process involves water heating a metre-by-metre thermoplastic mould which is then placed over the entire head and the shoulders. Breathing holes are cut out at the nose and the mouth by one nurse whilst the other sculpts the mould closely around the facial features before the mould hardens beyond manipulation.

It was a strange feeling having a large sheet of warm jelly draped over my face and shoulders. Actually, it was quite lovely, almost comforting, like a spa treatment until I felt it start to harden and constrict. Bolted down, unable to move, see clearly or breathe comfortably, I welcomed the shadowy-shape coming at my face with a shiny scalpel, even though one slip could cost me a nostril or lip. After the mouth, nostrils and eyes had been delicately cut around, I waited for the hardening process to finish and for a brief moment, the thought that I was wearing some sort of freaky German sex mask took hold of my mind. I remember making myself panic, worrying that if someone did decide to darken my mask, I would be totally powerless stopping them.

As I was visualising kicking off a sex-crazed maniac, the mould had sufficiently set for the two nurses to unbolt me from the table. My sex mask would then be transferred to the radiology department for my radiotherapy treatments. With my mask fitting inevitably running over time, I was straight into a clinic appointment with a sarcoma specialist for my pathology results. Once again, it was disappointing news. The pathology results were still unclear and now that they had exhausted domestic theories, they were pinning their hopes on a U.S oncologist who was enjoying his recent retirement on a yachting holiday somewhere off the coast of Mexico. Until his return, the doctors were reluctant to comment on anything, so we left in a stressed limbo and me having bizarre, sex mask-related nightmares that night.

FOR CHRISTMAS, A couple of months earlier, my sister had generously bought two tickets to see 'The Lighthouse Family' in Portsmouth. Mum and I had spent many enjoyable, formative years listening to their CDs together when we lived in Devon, and as the tickets had been acquired before my diagnosis, it seemed like the universe had delivered the perfect distraction not to be wasted.

It was a small, intimate venue with a capacity crowd of about two thousand, wedged in like sweaty sardines. As the warm-up act went through their paces, encouraging the already enthusiastic audience to join in, I felt deeply resentful of their joyous faces, almost to the point of anger. Their smiles, their laughter, their years ahead. Even though the speakers were making our chairs vibrate, the noise couldn't drown out my incessantly distressing thoughts. It was a horrid sensation which I'd never experienced, or ever want too again.

By the time 'The Lighthouse Family' had finished 'Live again', my anxiety levels were so high I could feel my heartbeat thudding in my tongue and couldn't wait to get out into the fresh air. Despite it being a lovely gift and sound theory, the outing had psychologically wounded me. I no longer wanted to be around crowds or even people enjoying themselves. I didn't fit in with them; I couldn't share their joy, their optimistic care-free future and so I started to alienate and marginalise myself under the guise of self-preservation.

ON 02/03/20, WE were back up in London, still hoping for the biopsy results, but it was not to be. Interpretation of the second biopsy had been just as inconclusive as the first. As they still weren't sure about how vascularly aggressive it was and were worried about the disease eating through my right orbital socket and eye, they decided first to try and shrink it with 25 radiotherapy sessions, then surgically remove the tumour along with 5mm of the surrounding bone and tissue. After 15 minutes of elusive conversation, my Mum, sister and I made our way back home, feeling the frustration stir.

The following day something in me broke. Hours of mumbling through tears, sitting on the edge of my bed, and looking out of the window, feeling crushing hopelessness. Every appointment we attended, hoping to get answers, only saw us redirected to another department. If we asked oncology, they would tell us we'd need to ask the sarcoma unit and so we'd ask the sarcoma unit and they would refer us to the head and neck department or back to oncology. We had all spent countless hours online, unsuccessfully researching for any information on my particular sarcoma, and now one of the best cancer hospitals in the world was stalling, unable to tell me whether I'd be seeing my next birthday. And so, whilst Anton enjoyed the freedom of my double bed, I spent four consecutive nights on the floor, curled up in the foetal position, under a duvet at the foot of my mother's bed.

The 12/03/20 was the start date of my 25 radiotherapy sessions. I would be travelling up five days a week, Mon – Fri, for five weeks, and each session in the sex mask would take 15 – 20 minutes. At any other time in London, I would absolutely dread having to make that daily excursion, but as it was, Lady Luck lent me her velvet-gloved hand in the form of the pandemic. The start of my treatment just so happened to coincide perfectly with Boris's first announcement of a nationwide lockdown.

Charmian, my hero big sister, kindly took leave from work to shuttle me to and from my sessions at the Marsden, easing any worries regarding parking or unforeseen side effects. We would travel up the A3, listening to Ken Bruce's pop-master at 10.30 on radio 2, self-righteously casting aspersions on other motorist's validity for using the road. As the passenger, I had taken to dosing myself up on Oromorph and would either sleep or burble rubbish, occasionally joining in with whatever was being sung on the radio.

London itself was an eerie ghost town. The usually heaving King's Road was so quiet you could have been mistaken for thinking there had been a catastrophic nuclear fallout. I saw more urban foxes than I did people. For me, it was marvellous. Instead of appointments and radiotherapy sessions taking half a day, we could be there and back home within 90 minutes, saving oodles of stress, petrol and time. It felt like I'd been given the keys to capital with unrestricted, exclusive access.

After the eighth session, I felt the treatment's first side effects. The inside of my right cheek and the back of my tongue were exceptionally sore, and over the following few sessions the soreness progressed into ulcers. As my mouth worsened, my right eye and the tumour began to swell, fuelling further anxieties about future facial reconstructions. The more anxious I became, the more I isolated and withdrew, often failing to respond to well-meaning messages. I couldn't articulate how I was feeling. I didn't know whether I was dying and didn't have the motivation to explain it, or the knowledge to answer the inevitable questions. I simply did not know what was happening to me, either psychologically or physically.

By 30/03/20 my right eye had swollen to the point of closure and the skin beneath it had begun to crack and, along with the persistent ulceration, both corners of my mouth had split. I had also lost all my taste buds which made food textually and tastefully unpleasant. I remember trying a digestive biscuit and being transported back to my infancy and the first time I grabbed a fistful of sand from our neighbour's sandpit for an ill-judged snack. The scans revealed that although the swelling had lessened, the tumour itself had not shrunk. I was prescribed precautionary anti-biotic eye drops and eczema skin moisturizer before I left the Marsden, downtrodden and disinterested in the scheduled conference call I had with the nutritionist and dietician later that afternoon.

The conference call raised more prospective complications. Without taste buds and a sore, ulcerated inside mouth, eating had completely lost its appeal. The dietician voiced her deepening concerns about weight loss citing the possible necessity of a gastro-tube and refitting of the sex mask if weight drop was too severe or sudden, so issued a prescription of highly-calorific yoghurts to be collected from my local G.P. I was now in a precarious position where if the swelling continued, I'd need another sex mask, but if I lost weight in my face I would also need to be refitted. Painful, daily jaw exercises and forced swallowing were strongly recommended regardless of any weight fluctuations. Use it or lose it was their gloomy message. A bottle of red wine and several oversized slurps of Oromorph sent me to sleep that night.

On 01/04/20 my eye had slightly improved but the radiotherapy side effects had worsened. The insides and corners of my mouth were raw and were accompanied by pounding headaches and the occasional nosebleed. I also started losing hair from the treatment site which gave the impression that someone had comically clean-shaved half my face whilst I was passed out. But despite the physical pain, it was the psychological stress of what was happening that greatly affected me. With far more questions than answers and nowhere to find them, my consumption of wine and morphine had rocketed in unsuccessful efforts to keep my mind from obsessing over speculative scenarios. The daily phone calls with the dietician regarding my weight were a blur and my answers to her enquiries fictitious, frightened that any truths would ultimately lead to me being fed through a tube.

YOU HAVE BEEN WARNED

'Death is like the rumble of distant thunder at a picnic'.
– W.H Auden

TUESDAY APRIL 14TH, 2020, will be a date forever branded on my brain. It had been almost four months to the day since my diagnosis date, four months of uncertainty, and four months of pickling self-destruction. With three radiotherapy sessions remaining, I was holding on to the hope there might be light at the end of the tunnel. My face had steadily swollen over the previous four weeks of treatment and my skin had become tender to the touch. With food being inedible, I was surviving on regular liquid morphine hits, red wine and calorific yoghurt drinks a couple of times a day.

In the afternoon, I began to feel unwell, prompting an early retirement to bed and hoping a traditional good night's sleep was all the remedy required. Nausea had other ideas. Sleep was impossible, as was finding comfort of any kind. Twice that night I was forced to do the bathroom dash, and both times, despite the desperate bouts of retching, I could only produce a small eggcup of greenish-yellow bile. As I warmly embraced the toilet, wishing I could die, I tried to recall what could have caused this new world of pain. My eating and living habits hadn't changed in weeks, and my stringent isolation conditions ruled out Coronavirus or any third-person infection, leaving me with the symptoms and only plausible explanation of radiation poisoning.

Wednesday proved no easier. My toilet runs were fast and

frequent. Anything that passed my lips would be readily rejected, including water but more importantly, morphine, leaving me with no pain relief and my face screaming at me.

It was on Wednesday night that I took a turn for the worse. Unable to regulate my inner thermostat, my body was going through waves of temperature extremes. One moment I would wrap my duvet tight around me, freezing, only to throw it off, open the window and gulp at fresh air like I was drowning. All the while, my helpless mother watched on with increasing concern. We had been given strict instructions to travel directly to the Royal Marsden if any problem arose, but as I was feverishly adamant that they had poisoned me, I was pleading she didn't call. When my muscles started to involuntary contract and I began slipping in and out of consciousness, she made the 999 call.

Charmian arrived minutes before the ambulance, by which time all of my muscles had fully contracted, giving me the posture of a frail, arthritic 90-year-old man. With my eyes rolling, my mother answered the paramedics questions and, after hearing my case's complexity and witnessing my rapid deterioration, decided to blue-light me to the Royal Surrey. They carried me downstairs as if I was a cardboard cut-out.

I am lucky, no question, that I only live 15 minutes from the hospital but those 15 minutes on that Thursday morning seemed like an eternity. If it had been any further, or they had insisted on the Royal Marsden, I honestly don't know what I would have done. Being dead was developing into an attractive option.

But Lady Luck has a knack for showing herself at the most peculiar times and often when most needed. My arrival at A & E happened to coincide with a shift change and due to the time of day, the ER department was quiet, enabling me the undivided attention of staff to whom I owe a lifetime's gratitude.

In my lucid moments, I tried my hardest to explain that the bastards at the Royal Marsden had poisoned me and insisted they Google 'Chernobyl' and Alexander Litvinenko for a better understanding. I was outraged at the suggestion it was alcohol-related and in better health would have been asking for the doctor's rank, file and number so I could make a formal complaint. Once they had skewered me with various needles, my nausea slowly diminished, making me think that maybe they did know what they were doing. Out of crippling pain, I was wheeled to the recovery room where I joined two other lifeless bodies and a couple of floating nurses. As I was lying there with a drip in my arm, slowly regaining consciousness, one of the nurses drew my attention for no other reason than her seemingly pointless bumbling. I watched her drift between cubicles offering water and, on occasion, comfort and questioned the value and purpose of her employment. My thoughts on NHS recruitment policies were interrupted by a very sudden, overwhelming compulsion to be anywhere but there. I yanked the drip out of my arm and scrambled to get off the bed. The last thing I recall is my body starting to shake violently.

I came partly round to find half a dozen masked doctors working busily around me. An oxygen mask was being held tightly over my face as a torch regularly passed from one eye to the other whilst a man shouted at me whether I could hear him. The urgency of their work and my ignorance of what was happening frightened me. As my heart rate increased and alarms sounded, I heard a quiet, softly-spoken voice in my ear. The words were inaudible, but the soothing tone was the only calm in a sea of medical commotion. The relief of a cold, wet flannel placed on my forehead was one of the most comforting sensations I've ever experienced. When my eyes found focus, the first face I wanted to see was the one that had given kindness. As I gauged her relaxed features and listened to her whispering words, I realised that, actually, for the patient, my 'bumbling' nurse was the most important person in that room and how very badly wrong I had been with my premature preconceptions. Again, I shall remain forever grateful for the comfort she gave during a particularly unsettling episode.

Once stabilised and observed for a further four hours without incident, I was transferred to a recovery ward. Compos mentis but enduring powerful waves of nausea, I couldn't understand how my alcohol consumption had induced a life-threatening seizure. The visiting duty doctor confirmed my fortune to be still breathing, considering 'organs had been compromised'.

I shared my ward with three older men, 'The Captain' in the bed opposite, Roger in the next bed on the right, and a third gentleman next to Roger. 'The Captain' was a husband, father of two, adoring grandfather to 6, a Falklands war veteran, a charity founder and volunteer for the past 30 years. He had also been slowly dying for two weeks. It was late in the afternoon when his elegantly dressed wife who had been escorted to the ward by the chaplain, drew the curtain around his cubicle for the last time. Listening to two people who have been in love for decades saying their final goodbyes is nothing like it is on TV or in the movies. There was a tender, tragic beauty that can never really be transferred onto the screen, regardless of how good the actor thinks they might be.

'The Captain's' death perturbed Roger, of similar age, who had grown quite close to him over the previous couple of weeks, sending him into a silent shock. Roger was an avid gardener, a semi-retired pest controller with a Homer Simpson hue whose symptoms had baffled the doctors for weeks. His alarming appearance presented all the hallmarks of extreme jaundice, yet all tests had come back negative, leading to his perplexed doctor asking about the availability of 'House.' When the suggestion of Weill's disease had been raised, his doctor had laughed, remarking that he had never had a Weill's disease case in all his years and would wage his annual salary it was anything but. On the morning I was preparing to leave, his Weill's disease test results were delivered by the same embarrassed consulting doctor who promptly apologised and thanked Roger for not taking his bet.

The other gentleman was nearest the window on the right. He was the withered, thinnest, eldest and sported a thin, straggly, unkempt, white beard which he habitually stroked with his nail-bitten, tobacco-stained fingers. He was a loud, aggressive patient, ignoring reasonable requests from my two other ward-mates not to use such industrial language and to show the mainly Philippine nursing staff some deserved respect. There was one point where I was sure the police would be called as he demanded that his tomato soup be reheated, shouting at anyone who dared to look in his direction.

That evening, about an hour after the ward's lights had been turned off for the night, I started to feel the all too familiar nausea steadily rising in my stomach. As I began wriggling around on the bed moaning, concerned Roger next to me went to find the duty nurse whilst the gentleman by the window, clearly irritated that I was keeping him awake, yelled out the encouraging words,

'Oh for fuck's sake, can you die fucking quietly please!'

Those words were the last I remembered.

I vividly recall the same dark, cold, lonely nothingness that I had felt during the first seizure in the recovery room and the same masked faces busily working around me when I came round. Coincidentally, whilst the doctors were bringing me back, it had been the first time since my admission that my mother and sister were able to get through to the ward sister on the phone and were told, 'I'm sorry, no one's available right now, the doctors are dealing with an emergency. Please try later'.

The following morning, feeling a whole lot better, Roger smiled at me, 'I thought we were going to lose you last night. You were like a man possessed, from one of those zombie TV shows'.

Meantime the scrotum by the window picked up from where he was the night before, bellowing that someone had "fucked up" his breakfast order. As the ward doctors, sisters and nurses gathered in a large agitated group discussing how to handle him 'this time', one by one, their conversations fell silent. Bursting through the middle like a sharp spear came a purposeful, tiny, elderly Asian woman dressed entirely in black, reading glasses on, with her hair tied back in a rubber band and a plastic visor shielding her chamois-creased skin. She wore no identifying lanyards or wristbands and bristled with a tangible menace.

She was covert, as if from the hospital's special forces, ninja department. With a laser-like unflinching stare, she locked on to the dickhead by the window and bustled directly towards him.

For the first time in hours, his rantings and pithy demands ceased, almost as if someone had vacuumed the breath out of his lungs. Every step she took closer, he recoiled further back in his bed, pulling his sheet tighter and tighter to his chin. He knew what was coming. He'd been here before.

Along with her threatening, wagging, knarled, index finger came a terrifying bout of unknown dialect at such volume it made the dormant spoon on the bowl of his untouched cereal rattle. It was staggering to witness such non-physical violence erupting from such a tiny creature. Her reign of verbal fire continued for two or three minutes as a growing number of medical staff and patients pushing drips gathered by the ward's entrance. With a final flurry of blurred arms, she spun round towards the door, scattering fearful onlookers in all directions, all jittery not to be on the wrong end of that twisted, nuclear little digit. No one spoke for what seemed like an eternity, not even when the visibly shaken alcoholic let out a usually hilarious high-pitched comedy fart.

The ward's tense atmosphere only lifted when a member of the catering staff, who was clearing away breakfast and had missed the most brutal bollocking known to man, remarked,

'Wow, it's miserable in here today.'

Half an hour later, a hunched porter arrived pushing a wheelchair and behind, the hospital's black-ops enforcer directing traffic with a series of guttural grunts and grave glares. She stood at the end of his bed, hands on hips like a steaming human teapot watching as he struggled to put his grubby jeans on. After his third failure, she lost patience, grabbed the jeans out of his trembling hands, and pointed at the wheelchair. Dressed only in his predictably ill-fitting hospital gown and faded blue, baggy y-fronts, he meekly maneuvered himself into the waiting wheelchair, clutching his balled, white tee shirt close to his chest. Once seated, she unceremoniously shoved his trousers into his lap, looked at the porter, barked a noise and pointed at the door. On the way out, she stopped, tapped the rigid fool on the shoulder and gestured at the two nurses who had been tending to him earlier. When nothing came, she tapped him again and projected such an ugly noise in his ear he cowered in his wheelchair and instinctively murmured a faint,

'Thank you…thank you for looking after me.'

With that, she pointed down the corridor and marched them off, clearing a path from behind with more aggressive, incoherent instructions and fierce-finger waving. Regardless of age or medical status, everyone understood and wisely moved aside as she made for the nearest exit.

On the afternoon of my release, I was more than happy to be leaving. Despite the world-class care I had received, the whole experience had been deeply troubling. Before my admittance, I had always been quite philosophical, even glib about death and had for some time harboured an unfounded belief that heaven and hell were contained within that moment of passing. A concentrated, emotional hit of all the pain and joy you had given yourself and others during your lifetime, letting you go with bountiful bliss or infernal anguish. The simple idea of being a good person with strong moral coding who would be rewarded at the end with a warm light and sense of 'golden piss' had always been a naively strong enough false pretence. Following the seizures, my existential fear of death remains a constant mental preoccupation. Whether it be elderly people or animals, dead insects, and on really bad days, fallen trees, strangled by ivy, can all have an adverse effect on me mentally for hours, but my hardest struggle is living with and watching the two souls I love most in this world age, and being unable to curb or slow that unstoppable, one-way descent to that cold, lonely, frightening place.

When I walked out of that hospital 72 hours later, I was a very different person from the one who had been carried in. Sure, I still had a sizeable, rare cancer growing out of my face, but there had been an unmistakable shift in perspective. I remember standing outside the hospital's entrance, waiting for my sister to pick me up, and in the likelihood of sounding clichéd, I viewed things differently. For instance, I saw the range of greens in individual leaves and the blue in the sky had a depth I hadn't noticed before. They'd always been there; I'd just never seen them. Even the yellow 'Ambulances only' written on the asphalt had a wondrous appeal about it. It felt like I had been reborn, or as if a spell had been lifted. I saw the world for the first time through new, sharper eyes. I had an almost canine sense of hearing and smell. The air was sweet; apart from the occasional whiff of the discarded burger and chips by the sliding doors; I heard a cacophony of deafening spring birdsong in surround sound. It was one of those precious mental snapshots that still serves as an effective under armour in times when personal peace doesn't seem possible.

As I was driven away, I vowed never to endure that self-inflicted pain again and decided to knock the booze on the head and stop using morphine as a means of recreation or distraction.

I returned home and immediately became aware that my experience had induced other unconscious transformations in me. For a start, some of my taste buds had returned, and out of nowhere, I suddenly had an insatiable appetite for apples. I'd never previously been a massive follower of the apple but I can only imagine the intense craving that I felt might be similar to pregnancy cravings. I'd devour any variety I could get my hands on from cooking apples to granny smiths to pink ladies. If it hadn't been for my mother's exhaustive trips to the profiteering local supermarket and sensible daily allowance, there was a strong possibility I would have been making an untimely return to the hospital with severe digestive discomfort.

My apple addiction lasted about a month, ending as suddenly as it had started, to be replaced with a determined compulsion to minimise and organise. Clothes, photos, letters, anything that hadn't been of purpose over the last year was ruthlessly discarded. I found I no longer had any sentimental or emotional attachment to anything, and every item discarded lifted a slight pressure. Even my grandfathers prized Mercedes bit the bullet. It had outgrown modern parking spaces and filling her bottomless tank cost as much as some people earn in a month. Her moods swings and unreliability were getting worse into her old age. Each venture had become a game of Russian roulette on whether I'd make it home or end up on the side of the road waiting for a recovery vehicle. Her next carer was an elated Irishman who had travelled over from Cork in a flatbed. As he handed me a white envelope full of cash, I decided not to quibble about the necessity of his trip in a strict lockdown and after one last quite word of thanks, wished her well on the Emerald Isle and waved her goodbye.

The belongings that did survive the culling were organised and reorganised, folded and refolded to the point where now, at 44 years old, I can get all my earthly possessions under my bed. On some level, I was preparing for my demise, getting all my affairs in order in one neat, easily manageable and forgettable package.

With my drastic downsizing, I was making increasingly frequent trips to the community tip, a mere 10-minute drive, door to skip. Parking the car up, I began making my way between the skips, vehemently sticking to the rigid guidelines that hung on swinging boards overhead. On one return journey, some mislaid pieces of polystyrene, stirred up by the wind, drifted untidily across the site, triggering my new obsession with cleanliness and organisation. No sooner had I started retrieving the stray debris from between the skips than a terrifying Lenny Maclean doppelgänger came bundling out of a portacabin and hurtled towards me. He stopped five yards away and addressed me in a strong Scottish accent,

'Oi, what the hell are you doing? Where's your hat and high-vis? No hat, no high-vis, no fucking job. Save your breath; I've heard more excuses than you've had solid shits; now fuck off and don't let me see you on-site again.'

Before I could respond, he turned, shook his head and disappeared back into the portacabin, leaving me in the curious position of being banned from my local tip and fired from a job I never had.

WHO'S A PRETTY BOY THEN?

'If the patient isn't dead, you can always make him worse if you try hard enough' – **Frank Vertosick**

Now THAT MY days didn't swing between nursing a hangover or earning one, I found so many more hours that I hadn't seen in years. Along with these new productive hours also came more time to think about the upcoming treatment plan and the potential aftermath. Without booze numbing the synapses, and aside from walking Anton, I had to find a healthy alternative to keep my mind distracted, occupied and so I plunged myself into mindfulness by taking up the challenge to fold 1000 origami cranes and as a small gesture of my enormous gratitude for everything she had done for me, promised my sister, Charmian, the 1000th. In Japanese folklore, if a person folds 1000 cranes in a year, they are granted one wish. I wasn't doing it for any fabled desire; that would be ridiculous, right? I was simply doing it for mindfulness, for good mental health.

With my 25 radiotherapy sessions completed, the next couple of months slipped past in relative peace and obscurity as we waited for information on operations. Days would be spent manufacturing as many paper birds as my patience allowed, often producing 50-60 a day. Whilst some part of me was driven on by the completion of the task, another part constantly told me to slow down and perfect crisp edges, apprehensive that once the final crane was born, I'd be left with a self-destructive mind.

On 29/06/20, we received the long-awaited phone call that the first operation would be 5 – 6 hours and would take place in a 'couple of weeks.' Despite finally hearing about the operation, the details were, at best, vague. The secretary who had phoned had been unable to answer the most basic questions leaving us caught in the cracks of three unwilling departments again, and so as we had many times previously, we rang the MacMillan hotline at the Marsden for information.

On 14/07/20 and eight long months since diagnosis, I went under the knife for the first time. It had been 8 months of not knowing whether the cancer I could see growing out of my head was terminal. 8 months for my mother to lie awake at night and plan her son's funeral. 8 consistent months of pain.

I woke from the operation expecting my head to be in bandages like the invisible man, but to my surprise, I was completely intact; as was the tumour. The operation had been a success in terms of preparation and also establishing the necessity for a more invasive second which had subsequently been booked for 11/08/20. The same disinterested French surgeon would be cutting from the middle of my top lip, up to the bottom of my nose, around the right nostril, up between the nose and cheek to my eye, and around my bottom eye-lid to the other corner of the eye. A flap, essentially, from which they could cut out the tumour and have a closer look at the eye and the bone beneath. Now that the surgeons had a confirmed course of action, I spent the lead-up attending appointments with various departments, including orthodontics.

Two hours late, the orthodontic consultant casually drifted by and asked me to take a seat in her office without so much as a hello or how's your father? She then spent the next half hour terrifying me on what to expect post-operation number two. My teeth and gums from the incisors back would be extracted. The roof of my mouth would be removed to access the tumour, where a bung would be inserted to fill the hole left by the tumour, which, for 8 – 12 months, would look like I had a severe abscess in my cheek, probably impeding my speech indefinitely. I would also have a temporary obturator fitted and was warned that everything I ate or drank would most likely come down my nose for the rest of my life.

'All in all, pretty horrible I'm afraid,' she concluded with a strange half-smile. She didn't know the future of my right eye and, until 'they got in', wouldn't be able to provide answers to how much of my face they would be leaving me with. I left the consulting room a little shaky, struck by the gravity of the news, the barbarity of the operation, and wondering what the hell an obturator was. It wasn't all doom and gloom though; at least I had Lady Luck to thank for the once-in-a-millennium compulsory face masking.

After consulting Professor Google at home that night, I learnt that an obturator is a '*prosthetic device that closes or blocks up an opening*' – *Merriam-Webster dictionary 18/01/23.* What that meant in reality and how it applied to me, I had no idea.

I spent my 43rd birthday having pre-op checks, getting needled by a trainee nurse and trying to imagine what my face would look like on my 44th birthday.

Three days later, on 11/08/20, I had my second operation. The relief of the wait being over far outweighed the fear of the surgeon's scalpel. Six hours after I was told by the jolly anaesthetist that 'we don't do pain here,' I came around in the recovery room. There had been no complications and the tumour had been removed successfully. Along with the tumour, they removed some diseased cheekbone and most of the orbital bone beneath my eye, leaving me a skinny, fragile ledge that did just enough to maintain structure. A temporary bung and obturator had been inserted, the flap replaced and stitched and for the sake of the stitches, I was enthusiastically discouraged from trying to speak.

After four days of being fed through a drip, I was deemed safe and well enough to be discharged with a large bag of medicated yoghurts. The once dream-like door-to-door commute time of 45 minutes seemed a distant memory as I sat staring at blurred brake lights for 7 hours following an accident on the A3, with no pain relief whilst the private ambulance driver babbled away incessantly on his hands-free mobile, wearing his mask as a chin strap.

I spent the following week in almost monastic silence, thankful for Netflix and looking like I had kissed a chainsaw. When I returned to have my stitches out, even I thought it a little premature considering my lip had yet to fuse but the nurse saw it differently and proceeded to cut the stitches out anyway.

I also had another appointment with the orthodontic consultant that same afternoon. The scribbled A4 piece of paper stuck on the door telling patients 'Back in 45' did nothing to soften my mood so instead of blankly staring at the wall, ruminating about my future, I decided to wait downstairs in the central atrium. Occupied chairs lined the sides, facing a grand piano in the centre. As I scanned the room looking for an empty seat, the female pianist jumped up and asked whether I would mind keeping my eye on her Sainsbury's bag-for-life, propped up against the piano leg, whilst she had a quick toilet break. Being the only cushioned seat in the room, I was delighted to oblige and made myself comfortable as she dashed out of the room and down the corridor. I hadn't been seated long when a little old lady, so immobile she would struggle to out-manoeuvre a wardrobe, approached agonising slowly.

'Do you do requests?' she quietly asked, panting heavily through her oxygen mask.

'I'm not the pianist' I politely responded.

'I'm sorry, I didn't catch that' she says, creeping closer.

'I'M NOT THE PIANIST' I repeat louder.

Nothing.

'PIANIST' I said, shaking my head, pointing at myself.

When her wrinkled face screwed up behind her mask and she turned away, it dawned on me there might have been a massive miscommunication. As my top lip had split, I couldn't form and pronounce the letter 't,' so all she was hearing was my pleading to her that I wasn't THE PENIS; perhaps too much.

No sooner had the offended old lady turned her back on me and hobbled away on her sticks, pushing her oxygen tank, the legitimate pianist returned.

'Thank you so much,' she offered as we exchange places.

'Right then, any requests?' she joyfully asked, looking around God's waiting room.

I left her to it and returned upstairs to the safety of staring at blank, white walls.

An hour and a half later, after a frosty reception, I took my place on the orthodontist's reclining chair, under the mirror and blinding lights. She totally disregarded the fragility of my bloody lip and proceeded to, one by one, insert wooden spatulas, similar to lolly sticks between my upper and lower jaws to measure my mouths aperture. My squirming and resistance were met with distinct disdain and strong, passive aggression. Still seemingly oblivious to my limitations, she gave me a small plastic bag full of spatulas with instructions to cram as many as I could until it hurt and then keep them in for 20 minutes, twice a day, for life. For the first time, the word 'trismus' was mentioned in passing.

At about 9 pm that evening, whilst drinking my evening yoghurt, my top-lip up to the bottom of my nose split open, leaving me trying to stem the blood with reams of toilet roll throughout the night. Early the following morning, we phoned the Marsden to explain the situation and express our desperation, only to be informed they didn't do emergency treatments. Terrific! We then sped to Haslemere hospital A&E who then directed us to the Royal Surrey A&E, who referred us back to the Marsden, who told us to sit tight.

So, on Friday 21/08/20 and after two days of looking like I'd been in a SAW movie, I was back at the Marsden to have my unstitched stitches restitched. As requested, I was in my ill-fitting hospital gown by mid-morning, in a ward on my own staring at the universal blue NHS curtains surrounding my cubicle. Seven hours later, I was still in my ill-fitting hospital gown, still in a ward on my own, still staring at the universal, blue NHS curtains that surrounded my cubicle, losing my shit. Apart from an insensitive offer of a cup of tea from a nurse, I hadn't seen anyone since the curtains had been drawn. Just as I was contemplating leaving hospital to find another hospital, a surgeon's green hatted head appeared around the curtain and no sooner had I seen him than he disappeared, leaving it to the nurse to throw herself on his grenade and tell me he wouldn't be stitching my lip because his 2-second examination from afar, suggested an infection. I wholeheartedly disagreed and angrily 'suggested' it was Friday afternoon, and he habitually had sex with his hand. I wasn't best pleased.

Stuck in Friday night traffic on the Kings Road trying to get home, lip split, quietly fuming, my mother and I received an emotional telephone call from the same nurse who had removed my stitches in the first place, apologising profusely for the wasted day and the shoddy treatment. Despite the good intention, the call only went so far in fuelling an already raging fire.

By 24/08/20, I'd had enough of the Marsden's aftercare and my lip hanging open, so phoned my GP to request a transfer of care to the Royal Surrey. As I was in limbo between the two hospitals, I wasn't sure who to contact for a repeat prescription of Pregabalin. As my supply dwindled and the weekend loomed, I didn't think three or four days of going without a dose would be a problem. How wrong I was. By Sunday afternoon, the itch in my face was driving me insane. Literally insane. I'd never thought that an un-scratchable irritation beneath the skin could cause such mental distress. One last crazed ruffle through my hospital belongings unearthed a stray capsule stuck inside my toiletry bag. 20 frightful minutes later, the worst of it had subsided, postponing the need of the steel wool I had taken from the kitchen sink. The whole episode graphically demonstrated my reluctant dependency on prescribed pain-killing medication.

The following morning, I was first in the queue waiting for the surgery to open, absolutely terrified not to go through another unmedicated ordeal like that again, all avoidable and solely down to my own disorganised stupidity. On leaving, the receptionist informed me that my transfer request to the Royal Surrey had been successful.

Although the Royal Surrey would take on my aftercare, I still had to attend sarcoma and oncology outpatient appointments at the Marsden until it had been determined that I no longer required further treatment. I was dreading the first post-surgery appointment I had with the arrogant French prick who had cut my face up and in expectation of going toe to toe with him, spent my time in the waiting room repetitively telling myself I was a tiger.

He disarmed my beast mode immediately by inviting me into the consulting room with such a changed, graceful demeanour I had to pinch myself and stop imagining he was taking me to a VIP table at the Moulin Rouge. He was the closest I've ever come to meeting a real-life Dr Jekyll and Mr. Hyde. He was charming, informative, patient, and I think I even detected some empathy. In amongst his sudden simplified medical jargon and sympathetic enquiries, he gave a worryingly detailed explanation of 'trismus,' or 'lockjaw' in common parlance. I had always assumed that 'lockjaw' was a symptom of tetanus that modern medicine had eradicated.

'Trismus, also called lockjaw, is a painful condition in which the chewing muscles of the jaw become contracted and sometimes inflamed, preventing the mouth from fully opening. Problems include feeding and swallowing, oral hygiene issues, and even difficulty speaking. Trismus may also last longer and could be more resistant to conventional treatment in those who develop fibrous tissue due to radiation therapy. Tumours that interfere with the function of the jaw itself can lead to trismus. But it more commonly occurs due to radiation of cancer involving the jaw. This can cause damage and lead to the creation of scar tissue around the joint area…' – www. healthline.com (02/07/22)

His advice on regular stretching with the wooden spatulas fell in line with both the orthodontic consultant's and dietician's recommendations, but when quizzed on how the fuck I was supposed to do the exercises with my face flapping open, he wasn't so forthcoming. But, regardless of my testy attitude, he remained remarkably composed. Everything made sense when he casually dropped into the conversation that he had received a phone call from my concerned G.P. the previous day. My G.P.'s fantastic but fearsome and even as a long-standing patient I'm terrified of her so God only knows what size arsehole she ripped him. Anyway, I left the appointment and hospital still requiring stitches, thinking that my aftercare wouldn't be as straightforward as I had hoped.

On 04/09/20, we received another disappointing phone call from the Marsden, delaying my restitching until 15/09/20, almost a month after they had come undone. By now, the two exposed sides of my wounded top lip were beginning to heal, giving me the attractive appearance of having two distinct top lips. Out of options, an urgent private appointment was reluctantly booked with the head and neck oncology consultant at the Royal Surrey.

Meanwhile, an infection had started to swell my face rapidly. The puce, red skin over the temporary bung had stretched so tautly that the surface had developed a sheen. And with it came a new form of chronic, physical pain, the likes I hadn't experienced before. My misdiagnosed broken/dislocated shoulder, the tropical abscess in my arm, and even the stitches in my foot without anaesthesia had all tested my resolve, however, this was something alien under the skin, growing like another cancer. The Oromorph, which I had begun using again for anxiety, offered paltry relief and only seemed effective at lengthening the time I spent in the bathroom, sat on the toilet. Thankfully, my disastrous Devon escapade had taught me that if I ever required a serious, emergency evacuation, all I needed was a baked camembert washed down with several rum and cokes.

As the pain steadily increased and my need for relief became more frantic, the once laughable idea of self-surgery was becoming more and more appealing. Before I took a bread knife to myself in front of the bathroom mirror, Mum bundled me into the car and drove me to the Royal Surrey's A & E department.

With covid still rife, I joined the stretched, sorry-looking queue outside, wondering how long I could distract myself hopping from foot to foot before I took a doctor hostage and demanded a sedative. The booking-in nurse was unmoved by my agitated, tearful state, asking me to take a seat and nonchalantly telling me to expect a two-hour wait. Unable to sit still with the beads of sweat steadily tumbling down my forehead, I approached the booking-in nurse again. Her earlier compassionate spirit somewhat diminished on seeing me a second time.

'I'm so sorry. I know you're busy, but is there any chance I could get some pain relief?'

She looked at me over the rim of her glasses.

'So, you're after drugs?'

From my animated, crazed fidgeting, and gradually dampening t-shirt, it was a fair assumption to make, and strictly speaking, I was.

'Well, yeah, for the pain.'

She went back to her paperwork.

'Would you like some paracetamol, sir?'

'No. I need something a bit stronger.' At which point I became aware of a man standing behind me, patiently waiting, holding a jam jar full of ice and two of his detached fingers.

'Then take a seat and a doctor will be with you shortly.'

Right then, for a terrible moment, I didn't know what to do with myself. Honestly and truthfully speaking, aside from some particularly dark, depressive episodes, that was the only time I've seriously considered taking my own life. It wasn't only the gnawing pain but the overwhelming sense of desperate helplessness.

Knowing I wouldn't last ½ an hour, let alone 2 hours, I circled the room trying to find the exit and a permanent way out and was probably only saved from doing something stupid by my mother's face at the window outside.

I can't remember Mum driving home; I'm not even sure I was conscious. What I do recall is rifling through all the cupboards in a frantic quest to find anything remotely painkilling. Anything numbing. Anything to get me through. Pregabalin, Paracetamol, Ibuprofen, Oromorph, I even smothered my head with Voltarol, such was my state of mind. My perseverance paid off. Within the hour, I had successfully passed out and made it through the day, which a few hours earlier had seemed most unlikely.

The pain had dipped slightly below suicidal levels the following morning, allowing Mum a brief window to make a series of hurried phone calls. The Marsden's pain team had done all they could; I was taking their recommended maximum medication and as far as they were concerned, it was job done. As far as I was concerned, they were as much use as a condom in a nunnery. So as the days passed and the swelling continued to engulf my eye, the private appointment with the head and neck oncology consultant at the Royal Surrey couldn't come soon enough.

Walking into his office, and before I had even removed my mask, his words were,

'My God! THAT needs to be changed.'

I could have hugged him. Not only was the bung badly infected but also way too big. The appointment was going encouragingly well. His years of experience, patient empathy and basic medical jargon reassured me that he was the right man to be talking to. As the discussion progressed, and I vented my spleen, he asked me who had overseen my surgery at the Marsden. I had never seen a grown man's manner change so rapidly when I gave him my answer. Awkwardly, it transpired that the head of the department at the Marsden had been his mentor for years, placing him in a proper professional pickle. For a few moments, he mumbled and bumbled away as his cogs worked out his ethical position and realigned his moral compass.

Having composed himself, he was quite open in telling us that he wasn't looking forward to 'the uncomfortable conversation' that he would be having with his mentor that evening. My mother and I left with a hefty invoice but at last with the optimism that someone actually gave a shit.

I would have loved to have been a fly on the wall for that 'uncomfortable conversation' that evening because whatever was said, clearly hit home. Early the following morning, we received a phone call from the Marsden confirming an obturator change, a replacement bung and lip stitching to be carried out on 15/09/20. It was a rare day of celebration.

It was around this time, when out walking Anton, I came upon the golf club steward/cricket umpire ambling towards me. Without any escape routes, I had to finally confront the golf club ghost and braced myself for a verbal roasting. But it never came. His recent cancer diagnosis had softened his outlook as it so often does, and if anything, he had admired my golf-club heist. Although his prognosis was optimistic and treatment relatively straight-forward, we spoke openly about our feelings, fears, family and the future and by the time we parted, I like to think we had crossed the line from being acquaintances to being friends. We even agreed to meet for supportive dog-walks. It was a huge relief to have finally cleared the air and also to have found a support and an ally in the most unlikely person.

We never did walk the dog. After initially responding well to treatment, he took a sudden and ultimately fatal turn, sadly expiring weeks before his daughter's wedding, leaving behind an adoring, heart-broken family. I couldn't help feeling forlorn and guilty. He had many more reasons to be alive than I did.

THE AGONY AND THE ECSTASY

'The trouble with always trying to preserve the health of the body is that it is so difficult to do without destroying the health of the mind.' – **G.K Chesterton**

On 13/09/20, AFTER stubbornly and stupidly ignoring numerous people's advice and regular television infomercials, I made the long overdue phone call to MacMillans. Until then, my ignorance of the MacMillan charity was limited to thinking they served solely as a cancer counselling organisation that also assisted the Marsden administratively, so when a home visit was arranged for 16/09/20, I failed to see its purpose. I was in persistent, chronic pain; I needed medication, not talking therapy.

That afternoon, I shut the door on the world and worked my way through the last of the 1000 cranes. During production, I had often imagined the one wish the 1000th crane would grant me. As the months passed, so had my dreams for health, happiness, and a Greek villa with a swimming pool. For the last three hundred cranes, I had only one wish; to be pain-free for just an hour. An hour's respite from constantly and consciously wrestling to be mentally stronger than the screaming pain. Having exhausted all other pain-relief avenues, I had started to cling to the fantastical hope that maybe, just maybe, just this once, that one wish *had* to come true. I had nothing else left. Delicately placing Charmian's 1000th crane on the window sill, I primed myself for the lightning bolt of salvation. I still hadn't given up hope by bedtime and left my bedroom window open like a child waiting for the tooth fairy to visit. No-one, wishful or otherwise came to visit. If anything, the pain had worsened overnight, stripping the last of my strength.

On 15/09/20, we made our way back up to the Marsden to be restitched, fully expecting to spend the day there and then be sent home for some spurious reason or other. Unnervingly, everything ran to schedule. It was as if I was in a completely different hospital. The private consultation and 'uncomfortable conversation' were still paying off.

With the anaesthetist by my side, I lay on the bed in the pre-op room, trying to keep my dignity intact with yet another grossly under-sized gown and vividly remember the surgeon asking me how I was feeling. I just popped. Grabbing him by his gloved hand, I looked at him through tearful blurry eyes and pleaded,

'Please take the pain away.'

I vaguely recall him solemnly nodding before the most welcome anaesthetic kicked in.

When I came around, I immediately felt the pressure in my face had been released. The temporary bung had been replaced with a suitably sized one, my obturator had been cleaned and my lips stitched back together. It had been a truly great day out. As grateful as I was, I still didn't trust them with my stitches, so on my discharge, requested for the stitches to be removed at my local G.P. surgery, in full knowledge that anyone who disagreed would have to answer to my G.P. and be the unwilling recipient of a new arsehole.

When the MacMillan nurse arrived the following morning, I still held little hope of achieving anything worthwhile. That all changed within minutes. After hearing a brief summary, she was surprised that the Marsden's pain team hadn't prescribed Fentanyl patches. Without any further ado, she called my G.P.'s surgery and the Marsden to arrange an immediate conference call to discuss its usage. Although her visit was brief, it was the first time in a while that a medical professional was genuinely more interested in me, the patient and the life-changing injuries it would leave behind than the cancer. She had empathy. She listened. She cared. She emphasised how MacMillan is holistic and supports anyone directly or non-directly affected by cancer. It felt as though she had opened a door for me.

Later that same afternoon, I received a phone call from the G.P.'s surgery informing me that my prescription was ready to pick up. Within 20 minutes, I had the first patch on my arm. Within an hour, I was virtually pain-free, going from a 9/10 on the pain scale to a 2/10. Not only did the patches provide physical relief but also substantial psychological relief. A deep, heavy sadness that I hadn't been aware of lifted, and now that I wasn't spending my waking hours ceaselessly trying to contain and control the pain, I found myself far more energised and with greater and clearer mental capacity. After months of debilitating pain and almost exactly 48 hours after I had folded Charmian's 1000th crane and made my wish, it had been realised. I kept the remaining 999 cranes and have them neatly folded in rows in a bulbous fish bowl as a reminder of the pain, but more importantly, as a reminder of the blissful alleviation.

If I had any other cancer diagnosis, MacMillan would be the first phone call I would make, my first port of call on what will be a very bruising sea. Not only did they hold my hand throughout the rest of my cancer by liaising with the various hospital departments and G.P.s, but they also provided equally vital aftercare counselling.

The next couple of weeks were euphoric. Despite barely leaving my room, I felt like I was on the greatest holiday of my life. You can keep your private island with helipads and celebrity chefs, nothing will or can ever better the time when Thames Water tasted like Dom Perignon, and bubbles in the bath became childishly amusing again.

September had started with an indefinite, painful future and ended with what should have been one of the best days of my life. On 28/09/20, I was back at the Marsden for another outpatient appointment. I was suspicious and honoured in equal measure that the French surgeon had found the time to see me. I hadn't forgotten the numerous times and months he had redirected all and every worrying question and concern to…well, anyone but him, so his forced, flickering smile and piss-warm reception were treated with modest hostility and a healthy dose of scepticism. I declined his invitation to take a seat, instead choosing to stand, arms crossed and listen impatiently to what he had to say, readying myself for the inevitable side-stepping that was bound to follow.

'I have good news, Mr Dobson; you longer require any further treatment.'

Now it made sense why he had gifted me his time. His look suggested I should get on my knees and thank him personally. When I was unmoved by his searching appreciation, he repeated himself,

'It's good news, Mr Dobson; you no longer require any further treatment.'

I removed my mask, pointed to my stitched lips, closed eye, severe swelling, temporary obturator, potential facial reconstruction and mouth just wide enough to word,

'What the fuck are you talking about?'

His biblical father-figure arrogance swiftly crumbled away as he checked his watch, told me it had been a pleasure seeing me, left the room and closed the door behind him.

I left the hospital with conflicting emotions. It had been nine months, two weeks since diagnosis and I should have been jubilant to hear the news I was in remission, but as for 'no longer require any further treatment' when my head looked like a rotting potato, that just angered me. I understand it's their job to rid me of cancer, and for that, I am eternally grateful, I am, but it seemed to me he had forgotten there was also a person attached to it.

As the days passed, I mellowed. I actually looked forward to my daily trips to have my stitches out one by one. Each stitch removed put the cancer further behind me. When my face eventually settled down and my eye reopened, I started to believe that maybe I wouldn't terrify everyone under the age of 12 with my year-round, permanent Halloween appearance. My mouth had stopped shrinking to the point where I could just about fit an end of a finger in and my facial hair had sporadically started sprouting again, covering unsightly scarring. The C word was used less frequently, and we, as a family, had a revived sense of optimism.

It didn't last long, however.

On 13/10/20, two weeks after I was given the all-clear, my sister Charmian was diagnosed with breast cancer.

Lady Luck had dealt us a cruel, low blow.

Extraordinary as the timing was, there was one, very thin, silver-lining though, if there ever can be with such unsettling news. Almost a year earlier, my diagnosis had sharply focused my sisters mind to the fragility of life and being the owlish thing that she is, had taken out insurance against similar misfortunes happening upon her. Her soothsaying and pragmatism were rightly and richly rewarded with a generous recompense you would expect from such unlikely odds.

With cancer back in our lives, it dominated conversations, threatened future plans and cranked up anxiety levels. It mentally regressed me to the time of my diagnosis and the sadness, loneliness and pain that followed. I started to psychologically unravel. At times, I questioned whether I was being punished for breaking my oath of religious servitude I made to God if he helped me beat Glenn York in my maths exam when I was 7.

By the time I had my inaugural telephone counselling session on 22/10/20 with a MacMillan counsellor, I was broken. The 50-minute call primarily consisted of sobbing and snotting into my own quivering hands. Nevertheless, just having the opportunity to unburden such overwhelming emotions was a profoundly cathartic, soulful cleansing and just as valued, if not more so than any medicated analgesic.

Over the next few wintering weeks, I hid away in my room, staring back out of my window at the trees I knew so well, gripped by a merciless melancholy, counting down the days and hours until I could sob down the phone to a faceless stranger. Every call released pressure, just enough to keep me safe and sensible without needing a blood-let until the next weeks call.

My self-imposed isolation and withdrawal only fed the growing black dog, but it was different this time, a different breed. Instead of a persistent nagging and yapping trying to undermine and wear down resilience, this dog was bigger, growled a deeper growl and I was just as powerless. Rather than the thousand negative thoughts I usually have to sift through to find one positive; this dog gave me one immovable, blanketed conviction that consumed all feelings and ponderings, day and night with fluctuating waves of intensity. Try as I might, I couldn't shake the dog's unrelenting conviction that I *will* die alone and lonely. Outings had become exclusively for medical purposes. I was either going to my GP for medication or blood tests or travelling to the Royal Surrey to see the restorative dental consultant to get a permanent obturator measured and fitted. As he candidly said on my first visit,

'we're going to get to know one another.'

He wasn't wrong.

CHRISTMAS 20/21 WAS truly unremarkable. It was so unremarkable I cannot recall one day. It's no ground-breaking revelation that the winter months make perfect bed-fellows with depression, but none more so than the 20/21 winter of my discontent. My daily mouth stretches with the lolly sticks and the effort of eating was gradually eroding my quality of life and optimism. The weekly appointments with the orthodontic consultant at the Royal Surrey had become tedious, routinely painful and inevitably late, not that the waiting bothered me; I was always genuinely grateful to be seen whenever it was. For my new bespoke obturator, accurate impressions of the inside of my mouth had to be taken, and then sent off to the manufacturing labs. The problem was, I could only open my mouth ¼ of an inch. Casts were crammed in, impressed, only to be ruined on removal, rendering them useless and starting the process over again until time permitted.

On 10/03/21, I had the first NHS appointment with the 'private' consultant we had seen four months earlier. I'm not sure whether it was seeing him again or just my need to weep at anyone, but I was a blithering mess as soon as I saw him. Such was my desolate, desperate state, the appointment was a scramble of internal phone calls requesting urgent meetings with clinical specialists. With none available, scribbled numbers and business cards were offered along with the assurances he would personally be contacting my G.P. to express his concerns regarding my mental health. Neither my cancer nor my rehabilitation was ever mentioned. They weren't the priority. Stopping my mind from imploding any further was far more pressing. There wouldn't be any need for rehabilitation if I couldn't get through this phase. I repeatedly thanked and apologised for wasting his time, as I did the lady in the corridor, a hospital porter, and the security guard handing out face masks at the entrance. With my mother's arm firmly around my shoulder holding me up, she led me to the car, belted me in and drove home. The outing was a brutal illustration of my ruptured state of mind and reinforced the thought I wasn't well enough to be around or have contact with people.

In the few fleeting moments when the cancers side-effects weren't all-consuming, or the growling too deafening, I had started thinking of Jenny. She had been my ever-present best human friend since Wee-man had found his god in the hills of California years earlier. I had missed her and our friendship sorely, and the more I thought of her, the more I missed her. By this point, I had almost entirely removed myself from society, turning my phone off and only very seldomly seeing friends, usually by accident rather than design. During these rare, brief encounters, I had learnt that Jenny was in a relationship, and despite being genuinely happy to hear the news, hoping that she had found someone who deserves her, it only stiffened the black dog's claim that I'd die alone, spiralling me down further. When I hit my lowest point, I finally turned on my phone and made contact, arranging to meet Jenny on one of her mid-week dog walks.

I agonised for hours over my two aftershave choices, and went through dozens of clothing and shoe combinations in front of the mirror, all the while standing so that the right side of my face was always partially shadowed. When the day arrived, the only colour I felt comfortable in, was black, from head to toe and despite the unseasonably warm day, included a black scarf for my facial insecurity rather than for its intended purpose. My levels of anxiety were barely tolerable as I waited for her van to pull into the car park and even though I hadn't seen Jenny for months, and everything about this rendezvous had been meticulously planned, I hadn't accounted for my abject mental health.

As soon as I saw her van, I could feel a giant wave building inside me. By the time we were face to face, I was ashamed. Tears streamed down my cheeks, more snot ran from my nose and my conversation consisted of a series of whimpering's and monosyllabic grunts. The longer we walked, the more I buried my head in my scarf. I cannot recall a single word spoken on that walk and by the time we were back in the car park I was barely able to stand. Moving like an old man, staring at my feet and openly sobbing, I parted company with Jenny and retreated to the sanctuary of the car and sat there long after she had departed, dissolving into the steering wheel and berating myself for being a total fuck-up.

ASIDE FROM THEIR swift, decisive action sourcing much-needed Fentanyl patches, MacMillan were still providing an equally valid painkilling service with weekly telephone counselling sessions. My counsellor was a lady in her middle years and although she disclosed very little of her private life, she had a buddha-like warmth and wisdom about her. We didn't actually talk much as most of the session I would be chuntering uncontrollably, but when I was briefly able to hold a conversation, her sensitivity and empathy played a huge part in strengthening my resolve.

But sadly, all good things come to an end and so as my mental health slowly improved, I became more and more conscious of using up my Macmillan "credit" and thought that my counsellor should probably be someone's else life-line, like she'd been mine for so many months. Our final session was conducted much in the same manner as our first, with ceaseless tears, except the tears were of humbling gratitude rather than the result of a splintered mind in anguish. I can honestly say with my hand on my heart, those 50-minute weekly sessions were just as important and integral in my cancer treatment and recovery as the radiotherapy or the surgeon who extracted the tumour itself.

Being a depressive, I wasn't a newcomer to talking therapies. From the hours and hours of CBT homework to being called a 'spiritual crow', thousands have been spent on different approaches over the years, with varying degrees of success. One of the better ones, a psychiatrist at the Priory once said,

'You can get to a point where you've seen so many counsellors, you become one yourself'.

With that in mind, I was so struck by the immediate and lasting power of the MacMillan sessions and the skill of the counsellor, I started to feel that maybe I'd found a worthwhile purpose to pursue and so started exploring introductory counselling courses.

With the world still gripped by the pandemic, courses were exclusively online, negating any geographical or travel concerns leaving me in the enviable position of being able to choose whichever school of counselling spoke loudest to me. After extensive consideration and lengthy navel-gazing, I decided on a CPCAB accredited college in Sussex that taught 'person-centred' counselling.

There were twelve of us in total from a myriad of backgrounds and life experiences, all with unique reasons for being there but all sharing a common ambition, to hopefully understand how to be better versions of ourselves. Once a week, for 4 hours, we would digitally gather and learn how to be effective, compassionate communicators. Considering 80% of communication is body language, it always tickled me that all we ever saw were tiny heads in boxes on a screen and the occasional cat's balloon knot wandering past.

SUPERMARKET SWEEP

'I don't shop very well...I just see what I need and get it.'
– **Maggie Stiefvater**

WEEKS PASSED AND aside from my weekly counselling course and infrequent dog walkers, I would go days without seeing or speaking to another soul, preferring Anton's quiet company. When I did happen upon other dog walkers, my facial injuries have caused some bizarre reactions, with most doing whatever they can to circumvent me. I've had people, both men and women do hasty 180° roundabout turns, climb over fences and wrestle through thick undergrowth to avoid contact. On days when I have little inner mettle, it smacks, making me feel freakish and terribly self-conscious, but on the good days, the panic etched on walkers' faces as they try and find an escape route amuses me.

Apart from walking Anton, I spent most of my time sitting on the edge of my bed, staring out the window, trying to process what I'd been through and trying to come to terms with my villainous façade. I knew the trees so well I had affectionately named them and had, over time grown quite attached to them. I'd watch them dance harmoniously in the southerlies and thrash angrily in the northerlies. In winter, when they were naked and silhouetted against the iron-grey sky, it always struck me how similar their bare branches and sub-branches were to the inner workings of the human lung. There was even a pang of sadness and a period of mourning when the neighbours instructed tree surgeons to fell Otto, a young oak, and Betty the beech tree.

Realising I was developing closer relationships with trees than people, something had to be done. I needed to reconnect, to be part of society and have a sense of belonging and community, so Anton and I made an anxious yet all too familiar train trip into Godalming.

Trusty rucksack and sunglasses on, earphones in and my best friend by my side, it felt good to be out. It was mid-afternoon on a Wednesday, and in no particular hurry, we wandered through town, weighing up beverage options until I decided upon a coffee and eyed up the perfect table from over the road. As we waited for the lights to change, more and more people gathered to wait with us, and on the opposite side, tens of Godalming college students had quietly amassed.

Mothers with expensive prams and borderline road-rage jostled for position as the wall of students marched towards us. We must have been exactly half away across and right in the middle of the busybodies when I felt a tug on the lead. At first, I didn't give it a glance, thinking it was no more than a brief entanglement with one of the passing legs. The second, more resistant tug made me stop. To my horror, for the first time since I've had him, Anton crouched that crouch and dumped, smack bang in the middle of the road, and, as I hadn't heeded the first warning, he'd left a three-yard trail.

Crabbing from side to side with my arms extended, apologising profusely, I stood over Anton, frantically waving and directing feet around Anton's freshly made string of sausages. Earphones still attached, I swung the rucksack off my back and began frantically rifling for poo bags. With pedestrians thinning, I found myself on my knees, surrounded by queuing, impatient motorists. To my astonishment and unexpected delight, my fingers stumbled upon one rogue, lone poo bag buried deep at the bottom. With Anton pulling on the lead, I was operating one-handed, so as I bagged the final chipolata, I could do nothing to prevent the slow, terminal slide of my sunglasses down my nose and onto the asphalt. With the bursting bag in hand, I picked up my sunglasses and somehow, when I stood back up, had tangled the bag around one of the wires of my dislodged headphones. The increasing din of car horns made me panic further. In my frantic haste to get out of the road, I casually threw my rucksack over my shoulder, inadvertently catching the straps buckle on the thin plastic poo bag, spilling some of its contents back onto the road, and leaving the rest swinging unpredictably in its broken cradle. Making matters worse, a small collective of students, who had noticed my predicament, stood by the roadside giggling behind their phones. Without choice, I reluctantly left the fallen strays to their fate and inched my way toward the onlookers on the pavement, keeping a nervous eye on the occupants in their plastic hammock, teetering precariously from my entangled headphone wires.

I didn't see the funny side of the smattering applause the hilarious college students gave me when I had made the safety of the pavement, and by the time I had untangled the turds, I was more than ready for home. But before I could return to the safety of my bedroom and my trees, I had promised mum a Greek salad for lunch and so walked the short distance to the supermarket, discarding my earphones and Anton's donations in a bin en-route.

Keeping myself to myself, I made my way around the aisles, ticking off my list. On completion, I headed for the cashiers and passed the hallowed, discounted, yellow-stickered trolley. Right there on top, as if they were waiting for me, half a cucumber and a bottle of extra virgin olive oil for ½ price. I gratefully swapped them for my full-price items and carried on to pay in a far jollier mood than I'd arrived. 10 seconds later, I felt a tap on my left shoulder,

'Excuse me, but what the hell do you think you are doing?'

Standing behind me was a dumpy woman with apple-cheeks and hips wide enough to seat a farmyard animal.

'You just picked those out of my trolley.'

'Isn't that the discount trolley' I stubbornly enquired.

'No. It's mine, and that's mine.' She lunged at me trying to grab the cucumber and knocked it out of my hand onto the floor.

'What the fu…'

Whilst picking it up, I heard a voice behind me.

'Everything OK here?' asked the uniformed security guard looking at each of us in turn.

'This man is stealing from my trolley.' She pleads to him.

'I'm not. It's a misunderstanding.'

'Sir, are you arguing over the two items in your hand?'

'No, I'm not arguing…'

'Right, madam, would it be alright with you if this gentleman had…those…two…items?'

She looked at the olive oil in one hand and the cucumber in the other.

'No, of course not. It looks like he needs them far more than I do', she said with a smiley, piggy face.

A small crowd had started to gather. I'm sure I recognized a few faces, I could feel their eyes exploring my recent scarring, imagining how it might have occurred.

'Sir, I think you should pay for your shopping and leave.'

He watched me place them in my basket and then ushered me to a waiting cashier. Such was his mistrust of me, he waited until I had paid, bagged and collected Anton before returning to his post by the doors.

To round off my most excellent day out, I realised as soon as I had boarded the train that somewhere, during all the excitement, I had lost my train ticket which landed me a £20 on-the-spot fine from a merciless conductor. Such was my urgency to pay the fine before my stop, I completely forgot about my shopping and waved it a frustrated goodbye on the platform as the train disappeared off to Portsmouth.

ONE-EYED WILLIE

'One eye sees, the other feels' – **Paul Klee**

WITH THE CHANGE of seasons came another shift in perspective. I was slowly coming to terms with my new appearance and being thoroughly jaded with hospitals had, at least for the time being, dismissed the idea of facial reconstruction. I was still attending weekly appointments with the orthodontist, getting ever closer to my bespoke obturator. He had found a strange angle at which he could insert the mould, obtain a clean impression and withdraw it without being it spoiled, hastening the process considerably. With my mouth opening staying at ¼ inch, I had worked out which malleable foods I could and couldn't squeeze into my mouth through a process of messy elimination. Regardless of the foodstuff or how diligent I had been, remnants of any meal could be found all down my front, on the floor and so much around my plate, you'd think a stubborn toddler had had a tantrum.

I had even had 'the balls' to turn my phone back on, if only to contact Jenny exclusively. We were communicating regularly and as sorry as I was that things hadn't worked out with her partner, it felt thoroughly nourishing to reconnect with her humour, warmth, and selfless lightness of being. Over the weeks we grew closer until we were formally courting, out doing what couples do and happily so.

On 18/05/21, I woke to a golf ball swelling under my right eye, prompting an immediate visit to my GP surgery, who sent me to A & E, where I sat for 6 hours only to be told to return the following morning for scans. It was good to be back. Dutifully, I arrived early the next day and waited 7 hours for scans. I was sent home with antibiotics and strict instructions not to drink on them. I've had plenty of anti-biotics in my life so when the doctor insisted on abstinence, I gave her a knowing half smile.

'No, seriously, Mr. Dobson, don't drink on them.' I smiled at her again.

Three hours later, I wished I'd heeded her warnings as I watched the half glass of red wine I had consumed running down the wall onto the sofa beneath. I'd never experienced projectile vomiting before then, and I was just as surprised as my mother sitting on the sofa at its velocity and range.

Nevertheless, the antibiotics seemed to work and by the time I had my appointment with maxillofacial, I felt optimistic. The swelling had subsided and the sun was shining. The scans revealed what looked like 'moth-eaten' bone under my right eye, but as the Marsden was monitoring my remission, my scans had been forwarded accordingly and any questions or concerns that I may have should be referred directly to them.

When I wasn't staring out of my bedroom window or in the mirror inspecting my eye, waiting for my vision to blur, I was frantically googling eye patches. I had three different ones in my Amazon basket, a simple black pirate one for everyday use, a dandy silk one with a ruby in for those special occasions, and one with a creepy eye on to wear at night, just in case of burglars.

On 07/06/21, I was back making the sickening journey back up the A3. Long gone were the days when I had VIP access to central London; I was back to being Joe Public, queuing at every opportunity and watching people walking into lampposts, glued to their phones. I was seen by the sarcoma specialist, who, having seen my scans, couldn't be sure of the cause of the swelling. She helpfully narrowed it down to three possibilities, osteomyelitis, osteo-radio necrosis or bone metastasis, but until more relevant eyes had poured over the images, she could neither confirm nor deny any diagnosis. She threw one last spanner in the works before she left. The best-case scenario, it was an isolated infection, but even if it was, how had it managed to get into the diseased site. The telephone consultation booked in a week's time would hopefully provide some answers, although past experience had taught me not to hold my breath. Speaking of breath, it had properly been knocked out of me and I felt as if I was back to square one, wondering whether the cancer was back, ravishing my head and face again, and if so, how urgently I should order the eye patches.

The telephone conversation a week later was a mixed bag. Thankfully there was no sign of the disease and I would be keeping my eye, but they were still at a loss as to how and why the infection had manifested in the first place. Until the infection had disappeared, I was to continue with the projectile vomiting antibiotics.

Meanwhile, my relationship with Jenny was slowly deteriorating, through no fault of hers but rather due to my own insecure inadequacies. A daily medicated cocktail of 300mg of Pregabalin combined with 300mg of Quetiapine and 450mg of Venlafaxine had rendered my libido pretty much obsolete, and being unable to open my mouth, prevented any form of bonding, intimacy or hot-blooded passion. Despite Jenny's sympathetic protestations, my sexual failings gradually wore away my confidence in being a legitimate lover and partner. The nights were the worst. Every time I climbed into bed, guilt and self-loathing made me choke during my incessant, tearful apologies. And so, on 08/07/21, in a regrettably selfish act, I decided to hurt one of the sweetest, most loving, and best friends I've ever had by feebly sending her a WhatsApp voice message asking for a 'friendly' relationship. To try and ease my shame and guilt, I had hoped to convince myself that I had done it for the benefit of Jenny, so that she could find someone who didn't have so many deeply-rooted physiological flaws, but nothing could forgive sending a voice message. My sense of shame was only strengthened later that day when I listened to her accurate analysis of me being a spineless shit and treating her like one too. She expressed her points colourfully, concisely and without reservation, leaving me in total agreement with what she had to say. Fearful of hearing further ugly truths, I timidly shut down my mobile, reassuring myself that my new ethos of 'if I'm not in people's lives, I can't disappoint them', would protect others from me.

On 13/07/21, I had a follow-up CT scan at the Marsden. I thought I knew all the radiographers so I was slightly surprised when an unknown, cheery, middle-aged woman collected me from the waiting room and led me to the dressing room. Removing my belt had sufficed for all my previous appointments, but I obeyed her instructions, removing my clothes and donning yet another child-sized gown.

It wasn't until I was wriggling around on the scanning table that a voice came through the speakers,

'Um… it's just a routine head and neck scan.'

The lady stopped lining me up for the machine and smiled,

'Would you bear with me for a moment, Mr. Dobson…arms down by your side please, legs shoulder width apart. Wider… wider…that's better.'

With that, she circled around and left by a door next to a blacked-out window. Seconds later, she came rushing back in and swung my feet off the table, apologising profusely.

'I'm so sorry…if you'd like to get dressed, Mr. Dobson and we'll try that again.'

Whilst I sat in the dressing room trying to unpick the gown's knotted cords, it dawned on me why she was so apologetic and eager to get me off the table. As I had been readjusting myself, the blackened window and eyes behind it, facing the soles of my feet, had quite literally a ringside view. If I'd known, I would have asked them to warm the table.

FOR RICHER AND FOR POORER

'The massage not only has excellent physical effects but also helps with bonding and is a way of showing affection'.
– **Francesca Gould**

THE LAST COUPLE of years had been challenging for all concerned but especially for mum who had had to bear the brunt of my various meltdowns, anxieties and pains. It's so much harder for loved ones watching on from the side-line than it is for the patient, and in testament to mum's incredible inner strength, she had maintained an unwavering stoicism throughout, but sharing your child's burden inevitably becomes emotionally and psychologically wearing, so when my sister suggested mum and I booked a break away at Boringdon, a spa hotel in Devon, it sounded perfect.

As the summer months drifted by and our much needed escape drew ever closer, the absence of Lady Luck in my life made me nervous. Four weeks before our getaway, she reappeared with all her bells and whistles, making August memorable for all the wrong reasons.

August 8th, my 44th birthday and a special one mainly because I had a heartbeat. Whilst my recovering sister, her new husband, mum and I were raising a glass to life and good health, the phone rang. Just when I thought I'd had all the day's presents, Lady Luck gave me hers. On the other end of the phone was my uncle tearfully informing us that my cousin Kim had been found dead alone in his house. It was a sad end for someone who had endured an equally sad life and in the space of 90 seconds, we went from toasting life to toasting *a* life. The black dog began growling again in the background.

Sunday, August 29th, President's Day at my beloved Witley cricket club, and another special date. After years of bowling my bollocks off, I was finally handed every discerning cricketer's holy grail, the hallowed W.C.C baggy, a cap bestowed to players for an outstanding, usually match-winning performance. Wearing my baggy proudly like a coronation crown and with my belly full of potato salad, I wobbled home in high spirits. When the front door opened, my victorious grin met mum's solemn grimace. Baboo, our beautiful Frankenstein cat had sadly used his 9th life on a road nearby. It was heart-breaking for both of us. Again, it had been a special day of polarising emotions. My baggy no longer represented a proud sporting achievement but serves only as a memory of the day we lost our dear Baboo.

A week later, on September 6th, it was Kim's funeral. He had lost his loving mother suddenly, in his late teens, and his only sister, Paula to Australia. As my uncle was too wounded, and Paula was unable to travel due to Australian covid restrictions, my sister Charmian bravely agreed to step-up and read Paula's gut-wrenching homage to her late brother. As hard as I fought, I couldn't help thinking that I could and maybe should be lying in that coffin and my sister Emma, in Australia, would be asking someone else to read her final words to me.

The following day we packed the car for Boringdon in sombre mood. While the 288 days I had spent as a cancer patient had been emotionally attritional, that August had been an unpleasant punchbag of extremes.

The health benefits were felt almost immediately into our 3½ hour southwest run to the sun. I can vividly recall passing Popham airfield on the A303, and for the first time in months, I felt I could breathe, as if Lady Luck had lifted her stiletto off my chest.

Situated on the outskirts of Dartmoor, not far from Plymouth, lies the beautiful Elizabethan Manor House of Boringdon. It is steeped in colourful history and retains many of its original features, including 'the secret bar', accessed only by pulling the correct book in an unassuming bookcase, and the 'Great Hall' with its enormous roaring fire and musicians gallery. It's a luxurious step back in time. More often than not, its impressive spa is populated with small cohorts of leisure ladies dressed in white-dressing gowns and matching towel turbans that float around like pockets of fluffy clouds, alternating between the pool's edge and the sun-trapped patio, sipping on iced, cucumber water, trading tall tales of their child's precocious genius and recommending extravagant island retreats with private butlers.

I'd seen my fair share of strangers in dressing gowns over the two previous years and so feeling adventurous, I left the sumptuous grounds of Boringdon and headed for a nearby, terraced pub we'd seen on the drive-in. The rusted scaffolding and blue graffiti did nothing for its aesthetic appeal. Nevertheless, the chalked, chained, weathered A board outside advertised all-day food and a picturesque beer garden. The perfect place for a reflective lunch in the sun.

The barman, in his fifties, wore the kind of home-knitted jumper a distant aunt would send you on your 10th birthday and darting behind a thick pair of tortoise-shelled chipped glasses, one very distinct lazy eye, making meaningful eye contact nigh on impossible. He was charming though, welcoming me warmly to his pub in his broad Devonshire accent, as did the two old gents nursing their half pints at the bar, respectfully bowing their heads in unison. When I asked to see the food menu, he proudly told me there was no need, as he knew it off by heart, at which point he turned to two faded 80's KP cards of nearly topless ladies and said,

'On the menu today, we have salted peanuts and dry roasted peanuts.'

The two pensioners at the bar quietly chortled. Questioning

the hot food claim on the board outside, he told me they hadn't served hot food since the chef went to the local Sainsbury's; four years previously. No problem I thought, I'll skip lunch, get a pint and unwind in the beer garden. There was a choice of one lager and two ales on tap, with the ales having florescent yellow stars offering a 20p discount. I decided upon the safer, lager option and as I ordered, a hush descended on the bar. The two old boys looked at the barman, who looked at them and then apologised, this time addressing me as 'sir.'

'I'm sorry sir, but I should inform you, that's our most expensive drink? Are you sure, sir?'

I drew on my recently acquired online diploma in body language, closely regarding all three men in turn, trying to gauge their interpretation of what the word 'expensive' could mean, and steadied myself. He carefully dusted-off the branded glass, poured a pint, placed it carefully on the bar in front of me and drew in breath.

'I'm awfully sorry, sir, but…but that's £3.60 please.' he said, wincing, expecting a slap round the face. I'd been paying £6.70 for the same pint of Kronenberg here in Surrey and no-one's ever apologised for its expense.

My fellow drinkers waited for my reaction. I could hear the clock behind the bar ticking. The atmosphere eased when I withdrew my card to pay. While fetching the card reader, he enquired whether I was a new local or just passing through. When I mentioned I was staying at Boringdon, the hush returned. He quietly repeated 'Boringdon,' looking at the two locals who then repeated it back to him before gazing back at me. It was like a soft echo; a whisper in the distant trees.

Pint in one hand, Anton on the lead in the other, I asked as to the whereabouts of the beer garden. Delighted with the question, the barman lifted the small-hinged end of the bar and requested I follow him. He first showed me the obsolete kitchen, pointing out the pointless oven, toaster, dishwasher and then a detailed guide of the female toilets, the male toilets, the storage room and through a narrow, crumbling corridor, the stairs up to the garden. He stopped at the top of the stairs and sighed. The postage stamp garden was enclosed on all four sides by high, windowless walls of the neighbouring terraced houses. Brown, patchy grass barely covered the sun-baked, cracked muddy ground, and around the perimeter, broken terracotta flower pots housed long dead stems that wilted mournfully over the sides. Meanwhile, Anton had successfully located the only barely surviving rose and emptied his bladder all over it, surely extinguishing the plants last hope.

'I'll let you drink it all in, sir' he proudly said without a hint of sarcasm, turned and disappeared down the stairs.

I scanned the barren wasteland for somewhere to sit and was faced with two attractive alternatives. I either took my chances on the one rotting bench with its exposed nails or on the crooked swing that had what looked like, by its generous size, a prominent human stool on it. I found myself almost bewitched, hypnotised, watching as it gently swung to and throw in the summer breeze, more through surreal disbelief than dietary fascination. I stood in the end and wondered how long I had to be out there before I could return inside without appearing rude or ungrateful for the tour. Not long was the answer. In fact, such was my urgency to leave paradise I set a new PB in pint downing, a record not broken since my univershitty days. I politely placed my empty glass on the bar, thanked the barman for his hospitality and congratulated him on his magnificent establishment. He replied that I was most welcome and could visit the garden anytime I came by, which I assured him would be difficult to forget.

On my way back to Boringdon, I popped into the Nisa next door to the pub to satisfy my urge for a Curly Wurly. The thin, aging, grey-haired, blue aproned lady behind the till handed me my arse when I opened the door and mindlessly wandered in with Anton at my heel.

'Is that a guide dog?' she boomed.

'Oh, no, he's...'

'If you're not blind, you obviously can't read.' She said,

pointing at the sign that only allowed guide dogs. I hurried outside and lashed Anton's lead around a lamppost and went back in. Whilst queuing, three youths in their late teens, hands down their grey Adidas tracksuits and acting as if they were going to commit armed robbery, brushed past me.

Handing her my Curly Wurly, she looked at me.

'Where you left your dog? There be travellers round 'ere, and they'll 'ave 'im, quick as a flash.'

It was like a pantomime.

'You there…' she shouts, pointing at the youth behind me, energy drink in one hand, keeping his manhood warm in the other.

'…go outside and look after this gentleman's dog.' she yelled, eyes and neck veins dangerously bulging. I could have paid for my Curly Wurly by then and been on my way, negating the need for his services entirely. Instead of pulling a knife on her, he subserviently replaced the energy drink in the fridge and left the shop. To be honest, I was far more concerned with him stealing Anton than the possibility of a passing, opportunist traveller.

'You have to be so careful these days,' she tells me, scanning the barcode as I craned my neck to lay eyes on Anton.

I left the shop, Curly Wurly in hand to find the youth standing in front of Anton, with his arms crossed, like a nightclub bouncer, staring down anyone who glanced in his direction, pedestrians and motorists alike. He untied Anton, gave me his lead and then thanked me for the pleasure.

To this day, I don't think I've never been regarded so highly, by so few, in such a short time than on that brief excursion. I felt like a Spitfire pilot.

Back in Boringdon, away from the steam rooms, saunas, and crass social climbing, purposeful, uniformed massage therapists went about their brisk business, escorting clients to treatment rooms, releasing them an hour later with flushed faces and a bloated sense of entitlement. And I had booked to be one of them.

As I waited to be collected for my hot-stone treatment, vivid flashbacks of my last disastrous massage in Devon made my nervous stomach churn, so much so that by the time my masseuse introduced herself, I had completed two toilet runs without satisfaction. I was led to my reassuringly expensive treatment room with lavender diffusers, church candles of differing heights and the dulcet tones of South American panpipes, keeping one eye on my bowels and the other on my heart rate. By the time she asked me to sit down and remove my slippers, I must have apologised thrice for my inane prattle.

Unknown to me, the first part of the treatment was washing my feet in a bowl of warm water. Ever since I was bitten on the foot by a psychotic fish in Thailand and stitched without anaesthetic, I can't stand having my feet touched, let alone have someone kneeling; washing them in such a submissive, biblical manner.

Wishing it to be over, my masseuse inadvertently touched the scar on my sole, causing an involuntary leg contraction which ended with my wet, perfumed big toe kicking her hard in the shoulder. In my hurry to apologise, my foot came down on the edge of the bowl, flipping it and sending the water all over the floor and her kneeling thighs. Standing up too quickly, I caught my dressing gown belt between the cushion and the side of the chair, opening my gown and leaving the poor masseuse's face a foot away from my crotch. As I looked down, scrabbling to pull my dressing gown around me, my heart skipped a beat. I was wearing my only pair of boxers missing a front button, and as these things always go, my rascal had, of course, escaped. She handled it very professionally, 'it' being the situation, not my blind, new-born mole. Regardless of my plentiful offers of help, she insisted I remained seated as she went about mopping up the water with towels on her hands and knees. She must have grown weary of my grovelling and shut me up with one single, stinging statement.

'It's fine, sir. I've seen worse.'

I didn't know how to respond to that, so I sat there gormlessly, listening to the pan pipes until being asked to climb aboard the massage table. She left the room with the wet towels, holding her shoulder, to be replaced a few minutes later by an older, more… robust woman. I spent the remainder of the treatment convinced I was being vengefully burnt on the outside with the super-hot hot stones and on the inside, struggling to understand what she meant by "I've seen worse."

Aside from the restorative massage and the hours spent loping half-naked between different heated rooms, conversations with mum were dominated by Emma in Australia. I missed her. A lot. I missed my nephew and niece. A lot. So did mum. A lot. Sometimes, the missing was so wrenching I'd watch 'Crocodile Dundee' and reread their well-wishing cards that clutter my bedside table to feel connected to them on some level. Since Emma's visit, directly after my diagnosis, mum and I had harboured optimistic ideas she'd return back to the U.K, but as the months passed, hope faded. I found it increasingly hard to accept that she wouldn't be coming, and combined with the fear of a funeral similar to my cousin Kim, nearly all conversations, regardless of the subject, would be twisted and distorted until the Emma dilemma took front stage. Speculative scenarios would be recycled and thrashed out over and over, pointlessly and painfully.

In the rare moments that Emma wasn't discussed, thoughts turned to where we were in our own respective lives. Holidays and survival are excellent reminders of re-evaluating priorities. It felt like we'd been the devil's dartboard for last couple of years, and so instead of waiting for the next prick, we'd be proactive for once and make a positive, decisive change for the good. Whilst reclining in the crystal steam room, the decision was made to up sticks and move back down to the open countryside of the South-West. Whether it was fond nostalgia, the slower, gentler way of life or because I knew where to get a pint of Kronenbourg for £3.60, the move proved too seductive not to entertain.

But, despite the highly emotive conversations and the massage mishap, the getaway had been a total success. Although I had begun to develop gills and Mum-webbed feet, the marathon spa sessions and change of scene had been a timely Godsend. With a rejuvenated sense of purpose and lowered blood pressure, the five-hour car journey home offered plenty of opportunity to reflect on another memorable Devon exploit.

THEY THINK IT'S ALL OVER...

'The future is not what it used to be'. – **Yogi Berra**

BACK HOME, DRUNK and sober conversations continued to be governed by family politics and whereabouts in the South-West our next chapter should begin. One night, glass in hand and with the discussion taking its usual animated, emotional course, mum sent an out-of-character email to Emma to vent her frustrations and convey her anger at Australia perpetually taking family members from her. Both my mother's brother and sister, my uncle and aunt, had emigrated to Australia (my uncle returned to the UK) and now she was losing her daughter and grandchildren to the same country. Sharing in Mum's pain, I backed up her email with an equally acerbic voicemail, condemning me into making one of the biggest mistakes of my life. As each day passed, Emma's deafening silence made it abundantly clear that our ill-conceived, drunken mistakes had cut her deeply.

Having thoroughly poisoned Emma against us, we started on our next project of finding somewhere to live. In the 12 years of living in the Wormley wonderland, we had noticed a steady increase in traffic around us, especially the main road which had already claimed the lives of two of our cats and we yearned the peace and quiet the South-West offered. With Mum being gracefully retired and me barely earning, residing in the stockbroker belt in one of the most expensive council tax bands outside London didn't seem to make sense anymore.

But, with what the agent expected our house to be sold for, it became blindingly apparent that the castle, maintained grounds, and private river access would have to be realistically revised as properties within our budget still mostly had an outdoor toilet.

The bidding war for our house, with which the agent was so enthused, never materialised. We were told we had missed the eight-year high housing market by a month and despite several generous reductions, offers were scarce, as were suitable, appropriate properties in the South-West. After dropping the house price by 10%, we finally agreed on a sale and started panicking about being homeless. The marathon sessions spent scrolling through estate agents' websites yielded little; properties were just as expensive in the South-West as they are 20 minutes from London, making us rethink the entire move.

The day we phoned the agent to cancel the sale was also the day our new neighbours moved in. When a flat-bed van laden with plastic furniture pulled in, I went out to give the driver directions to the local tip which probably wasn't the warmest welcome to the neighbourhood. The furniture belonged to a couple in their early 40s and their year-old baby girl. As soon as we saw the baby, we hurriedly discussed whether it was too late to phone the agent and revive the sale agreement. Just as we were thinking a crying baby would be bad enough, we found out the mother was deaf. Don't get me wrong, I have absolutely nothing against audio impaired people, apart from when they're not wearing their hearing aids and shrieking down a slide beneath my bedroom window. Each morning, I wake up panicking I'm at Alton Towers. I haven't heard the baby cry yet; if it has, it's drowned out by the mother enjoying herself on the slide.

I've only seen the three of them outside their back garden once, during the late Queen's street party. Like many parents these days, their doting is bordering on oppressive, so when they sat the little girl on the curb to play with a dandelion to get a drink, it was a rare separation. I wasn't far from her, maybe five feet, and whilst I watched her innocently muttering away, taking great delight in the dandelion, the beer bottle in my hand slipped. Instinctively, I shot my foot out to cushion the blow and prevent it from smashing but only succeeded in mistiming the bottle's descent and volleying the beer bottle at the baby. By some miracle, it gently glanced off the top of the baby's head and landed in a large flower pot a couple of yards behind, leaving the baby looking up at the sky like Chicken Licken and me in grateful disbelief. I spun around, fully expecting a bottling of my own, but in a bitter/sweet moment, I realised no one else had witnessed the perfect Alan Shearer flick. Shortly afterward, the mother returned to reclaim her chattering princess and dandelion and disappeared into the back garden to enjoy the slide again, none the wiser.

On 13/12/21, I was back, reclining in the orthodontist's tiny windowless room with a bright light in my face and my mouth wide open at ¼ inch. It was my penultimate appointment with him and the last with my temporary obturator. Before the final measurements and mould were sent to labs for my bespoke obturator, he had one last root around. It's an odd feeling to have someone's finger roaming around your head under the skin. In my peripherals, I could see his finger moving under my eye and feel him running along my natural and artificial features. If anything, it was counter-intuitively soothing, not insofar that I would book weekly sessions but as a unique, one-off sensory experience, it was quite pleasant. He did wear gloves, I think. As intimate and friendly as we had become, I wouldn't miss our little meetings.

HUNG LIKE AN ELF

'The way you spend Christmas is far more important than how much' – **Henry David Thoreau**

BACK IN SEPTEMBER, my sister had pulled the plug on joining us for Christmas at Boringdon, citing expense as the reason. With the deposits paid in August, the prospect of celebrating Christmas in our spiritual home of Devon as a family was just the soulful medicine we needed. Mum and I's decision to go ahead with our Devon escapade wasn't received well, nevertheless, we packed our bags and the three of us made our merry way down the A303.

I'd never spent Christmas at a hotel so I was apprehensive as to what to expect. At least I knew if it all got too much, I could just pop down the road for the world's cheapest Kronenbourg and a packet of peanuts in a beautiful beer garden. During a brief wander around, it quickly became glaringly obvious that I was the youngest guest by about 30 years and any ideas of a casual Christmas hook-up were well and truly quashed. The previous two months of punishing daily workouts intended to impress my future bride hadn't been necessary all along. But, being the only guest that hadn't had at least one hip replacement did give me one significant advantage; the spa.

Access to the spa from the hotel involves climbing a towering staircase whilst wearing flimsy sliders and a dressing gown. As most couldn't walk unaided, it was a trek too far, leaving me almost exclusive access for hours at a time. It was rockstar living. In fact, I became so confident I wouldn't be disturbed that on Christmas day, I left my trunks on a chair and did a leisurely couple of backstroke lengths in my birthday suit. Feeling liberated, I then proceeded onto the sauna, where I laid out until most of me had wrinkled and shrivelled.

With a festive spring in my step, I pulled on my trunks and dressing gown and made my back down the stairs. Passing through reception, I was surprised by what seemed like most of the hotel staff milling around, smiling and giggling. Good for them I thought, getting into the spirit of things, and I would have kept thinking that if the receptionist hadn't called out,

'Merry Christmas, Mr. Dobson. Did you enjoy your swim?' at which point laughter broke out. I felt my head burn up in embarrassment.

'Yes, thank you…although I found it a little cold in there today,' which sounded more sniggering. I bade them a joyous Christmas and left reception cursing myself for not looking for cameras, which, I discovered on Boxing Day, were plentiful, covering all and every angle.

That wasn't the end of my blushing for the day. Having dressed formally, mum and I made our way through the hotel, widely bypassing reception, searching for the evening buffet. As we went, we remarked on how quiet it was. The hotel was nowhere near full capacity, but even so, it was desolate, giving rise to imaginative speculation on where the other guests might be. Mum opened the door to the 'Great Hall' first and made for the first person she saw, strolled up to him and casually asked,

'Excuse me, young man, do you know where the buffet is?'

He lowered his microphone, smiled and turned to his other four bandmates shaking his head. They each stopped playing and glared ruefully at us. With a certain unmistakable annoyance, the singer took up the microphone again,

'Does anyone know where the buffet is?'

As I was behind the huge door, I hadn't seen the hundreds of local people and hotel guests who had packed out every square foot of the hall, including the musician's gallery above. For the second time that day, my head felt like it was going to combust. Onlookers found it far more amusing than the band or myself, and amongst the laughter, arms pointed to the door on the other side of the makeshift stage. As mum tottered off to the door, I followed behind with clasped hands offering profuse apologies to both the bothered band and the applauding audience.

We found the superb buffet. It was an exclusively cold-cut meat selection. We're exclusively vegetarian.

Although it hadn't been the family holiday we had envisaged when we booked in August, that Christmas at Boringdon with Anton and Mum will forever hold a special place in my heart, not only for the mishaps but for the sight of Mum's relaxed smile which had been missing for months. If I had one regret, it would be not finding the time to visit the bewitching beer garden down the road to enjoy a £3.60 pint of Kronenbourg.

ALMOST FAMOUS

'Many of our problems are blessings in disguise' – **Leslie Stone**

On 10/02/21, I had my final obturator fitting. My brand spanking new chrome obturator came out of a small cardboard box, complete with a structural hard gum and inset teeth. With the chrome plate being thinner than the temporary plastic one, I could slip it in and out like a greased weasel. The 1mm reduction in thickness, although it doesn't sound much, opened up a whole new world of food for me. That gained 1mm has allowed me the luxury of using a teaspoon to eat. Soups, ice cream, and desserts were back on the menu again. After careful navigation and pained determination, I could also just open wide enough to slip biscuits in again. The feral food cramming had lessened, as had the volume of edible debris that surrounded my eating area after each sitting, much to Anton's dismay. In saying my deepest thanks and final farewells to the restorative dental consultant, his team and the Royal Surrey's superb aftercare, I'd be lying to say there was a tear in my left eye.

Apart from the surveillance scans every six months and the likelihood of further facial infections, that was it; no more appointments in the diary, no more tedious expeditions to London or fingers exploring the inside of my head but perhaps best of all, no more indecent hospital gowns.

Some things didn't change though.

It had been a while since I was fired and banned from my local tip, but as I continued to embrace minimalism and cast out my unnecessary possessions, it was time to return. Self-conscious and slightly fearful of being manhandled off-site, I donned my sunglasses, face mask and baseball cap, hoping my cunning disguise would be convincing enough to avoid detection or any banned watchlist.

I sat in the usual queue, readjusting my coverings, waiting for my turn to be interrogated by a barrier operative on my cargo. On nearing his hut, I could see he was a particularly friendly employee, engaging each driver with an infectious smile, offering anecdotes where he could, oblivious to the growing number of irritated motorists sounding their horns. After one final mirror check, I drew up alongside him, wound down my window and readied myself for questioning.

'Good afternoon, sir…'

'Hello there' I politely mumbled through my face mask.

There was a pause in time, a tense silence as if his brain was catching up, before he very deliberately snapped his fingers and pointed at me.

'Ah, I know you!'

My sphincter tightened.

'You're that bloke off the telly, ain't ya?'

My sphincter relaxed. Then tightened again.

'My missus ain't gonna believe this! You're him ain't ya?'

Before I could disappoint him, he darted over to the portacabin and returned with a phone, a scrap of paper, a pen and to a tirade of abuse from the potty-mouthed bloke behind me. Back in the safety of his hut, he leaned out, took a selfie with me in the background, and gave me the pen and paper. Just as I was about to explain he must have me confused with someone else, another lengthy blast drowned me out on the horn from behind. And so, with my anxiety building, and his expectant, excited eyes boring holes into me, I ruefully scribbled a completely indecipherable squiggle and handed the pen and paper back to him hopefully.

'My missus loves ya! She's gonna be made up! Thanks mate.'

'No problem, buddy,' I said, willing the barrier up.

Finally, up it went, and as I drove under it, raising my window, nodding and smiling politely, my shredded pride engulfed me like the ripped bedsheet I was there to unload. I've never emptied my car so swiftly or been so skittish, constantly looking over my shoulder for someone running at me, telling me I'm banned or worse, another mistaken autograph hunter.

I made two additional trips to the tip thereafter, each time approaching the barrier and its guardian with a certain degree of dread and trepidation. After my first bogus autograph signing, I was sure that he would either be too embarrassed to mention it, wouldn't recognise me or would ban me again, and to be honest, all of those would have been easier to live with rather than what actually happened. I pulled up at the barrier and wound down my window. A grin spread across his face; without a word, he was off again, back into the portacabin and emerging with another scrap of torn paper and pen. My heart beat faster. Sure enough, he pulled out his phone, lent out, took another selfie, and handed me the pen and paper. I had a dilemma. Either I came clean, embarrassing both of us, or…

'Mate, she loved it! My missus…'

'Oh good!' I said, staring straight-ahead.

'Can ya make this one out to my daughter? She watches you every week; she loves ya…Jasmin, or Jaz, with one z…'

I just couldn't. I'd let it go too far.

With the pen hovering hesitantly over the paper, I realised that I was going to have a serious problem replicating my original signature.

'Sorry about this mate, ya must get it all the time. It will mean so much to her though…I dunno; best wishes or something, ya know? Course ya do, ya do it all the time, sorry mate.'

I've only ever done it once before.

And so, with a trembling, guilty hand, I extended my best wishes to "Jaz," signing off with what little I could remember of my unintelligible, celebrity signature. As he thanked me enthusiastically and raised the barrier, the same fraudulent feeling engulfed me again. There was absolutely no way the signatures matched or were distantly comparable; even Stevie Wonder could have seen that. I slowly drove off, glued to the rear-view mirror, certain that as soon as he saw the obvious discrepancies, he would be chasing me down with a volley of profanities. My relief at watching him put it in his jacket pocket was interrupted when I heard a loud slap on the bonnet. Having been concentrating so hard on the scrap of paper in the mirror, I hadn't noticed another employee walk out in front. The slap I had heard wasn't him hitting the bumper fortunately but rather him slapping the bonnet in valid protest to my inattentive driving. As he stood in front of the car, furiously waving his arms around, offering driving tips, I raised my hands in compliant apology. It was then I realised there was something terribly familiar about his Scottish accent and foreboding figure. When he stopped mid-sentence and his eyes narrowed, I knew I'd been recognised. The generic arm twirling turned to focused finger-pointing and with it, language that should be illegal. He really didn't like me. As I double-checked the door locking system, my peripherals picked up movement in the mirror. Charging to his colleague's aid was my superfan, and as he loomed larger in the mirror, my fight or flight response system kicked into overdrive, quite literally. While fleeing, the car wheels must have come perilously close to testing his steel toe-capped boots, so the car received another solid slap for the second time in under a minute.

I left the tip with just as much need to visit a tip as I had when I arrived.

CASTAWAY

'I just need some time in a beautiful place to clear my head.'
– J.M Ballet

BACK HOME, MY counselling career had hit a bump in the road. Armed with a CPCAB level 3 diploma, my next staging post was a level 4 diploma and BACP registration. As I'd gained both of the previous certifications over Zoom, the prospect of attending college once a week and confiding in heads that weren't half an inch tall on a screen and attached to bodies, stirred the student in me. In a world where we'll be crying out for talking therapists, I was mystified at why so few institutions offered so few places and those that did were always heavily over-subscribed. I held minimal hope of gaining one of the sixteen places available at my chosen college the following September when the receptionist sending out the application forms laughed in genuine surprise telling me I was candidate number 89.

I was interviewed by an earthy lady in her late fifties who had the aroma of someone who had spent the night in the stables, and could have benefitted greatly from even a lick of makeup. Her fraying, almost transparent woollen leggings were neither professional nor flattering and her bare feet exposed yellowed toe nails with an advanced fungal infection. From her 'organic' appearance, I recognised her as the same interviewer as a peer on my diploma three course had colourfully warned me about. He had preceded me, being candidate number 72 and had fallen foul of her within minutes after disagreeing on why he deserved a place on the course and his misunderstanding on the symbolic importance of naming and growing a cactus by the window. But I needed a place. I didn't have time or money to sit around for a year as I waited for the next academic year to roll by, and even then, there would be no guarantee that I would secure a place, leaving me staring down the career barrel indefinitely.

Taking a seat opposite her, I could immediately feel my windpipe start to constrict as my horse allergy took hold. The interview started with the expected questions on the potted cacti by the window and which one spoke loudest to me. My hazy, cliched metaphor on how my stunted choice represented a difficult life seemed to impress her and progressed me through to the next round of enquiries based entirely upon Freud's Oedipus complex theory. Question after question on my thoughts on incest. She was old enough to be my mother. Bearing in mind the interview was for an 'experiential' counselling course rather than psychodynamic, she neither justified her sordid interest or its relevance to what we were studying. Her final question was whether I minded going home with glitter in my beard. When she thanked me for "coming", I left wanting, no, needing an immediate shower, not to lower my arousal levels but to wash off all traces of the interview. I felt grotty. I drove home thinking that maybe some of my answers hadn't been detailed enough to satisfy her and was absolutely sure I wouldn't be hearing from her again. When I received an email the following morning congratulating me on my successful interview, I regarded it as a definite sign I was travelling down the right track and maybe, just maybe Lady Luck was pulling some strings for me.

Two weeks before enrolment day at college, mum generously took Anton and me away for a week's holiday on the picturesque Isle of Wight. The 'villa,' which Mum had booked after innumerable hours of painstaking research, boasted everything you'd possibly expect, need or wish for from self-catering accommodation. Close, but not too close to the ferry port and trunk roads, with a waterside view and nearby nature walks, two bedrooms, a lounge with an adjoining eating area and a fully equipped kitchen. It sounded perfect, and we couldn't wait to recharge on our island getaway.

Sitting behind two retired, leather-clad, easy-rider bikers as they compared their engine modifications did little for the environment or our holiday enthusiasm as we waited at Portsmouth for the ferry to dock. Having boarded, we left the car and headed to the dog-friendly deck at the boat's bow. The serene waters of the harbour steadily gave way to overcast, choppy conditions of the Solent, and as Mum and Anton retreated inside to shelter from the buffeting winds, I remained steadfast, embracing the energising elements in a pseudo, Titanic moment. When I turned around, the deck was mainly deserted save for a lone small, black poodle with a red lead trailing behind it, wandering about on the far side. Just as I considered going to its aid, the boat rolled, instantly triggering the poodle to squat and evacuate. Mid-way through, a weary-looking old, bald man wearing a transparent plastic poncho over a blue shirt with the thinnest legs I've ever seen appeared. Honestly writing, I've seen bigger legs hanging out of a nest from my bedroom window. Fighting the wind, he and his twiglets made their way over to 'Pablo' as he searched for poo bags in his trouser pockets. He must have been a yard away when 'Pablo,' having finished his work, ran off, leaving the man yelling into the wind and weighing up whether to pursue 'Pablo' or deal with his aftermath. Decision seemingly made, his poo-bag gloved hand took so long to reach down, the three turds had caught the wind and were being blown about the deck like a family of spooked mice. Watching him chase and round them up was like watching city slickers catching oiled piglets. Although I felt I should go to his aid, it made for such compelling viewing I was spellbound. It must have taken him 4 minutes to capture all three renegades, and by the time he straightened, he was exhausted, leaning on the side to catch some salty sea air, shirt collar flapping. As the rain started to fall, an unimpressed male voice came over the tanoy system,

'Can the owner of a black poodle come to the stern deck please. You will need to bring disposable bags which can be found in all pet-friendly lounges. Thank you.'

The old man bowed his head, sighed, and slowly made his way through the interconnecting door into the lounge, poo-bag swaying from a clenched fist. As soon as the door had closed behind him, it was flung open again by a young girl making a hurried bee-line to the same spot the old man had just vacated. No sooner had she planted her hands on the railing, she technicolour yawned. Her first launch over the side was the most successful. The quick succession of the second and third however, were directly into a gust of wind, returning the contents of her stomach all over her trousers and trainers. The fourth matted her hair and covered her cheek. When her mother joined her upwind to rub her back, she openly sobbed. With the rain getting heavier and the direction of the wind less predictable, I thought I'd seen enough expulsions for the 1-hour crossing, joining Mum and Anton in the lounge and leaving the mother picking what looked like partly digested carrot out of her distraught daughter's fringe.

With an icy gale howling through the car, we drove the short distance to our 'villa,' stopping at the entrance of the road, which both the satnav and the host's directions were telling us to follow. The road ahead of us looked like the air force had been using it for munitions testing. Craters four feet wide and a foot deep riddled the broken tarmac for as far as the eye could see. It was a warzone. On the side of the road to the right, with a prominent buckled front wheel, lay the rusting remains of a blue Volvo estate.

Our progress down the war-torn road was so slow, we were regularly overtaken by ambling ramblers, all craning their necks to see if we were about to have a bumper ripped off. Finally, and with the suspension creaking alarmingly, a faded, peeling sign ominously welcomed us to our 'villa' or rather collection of 'villas.' On either side of a gravel track were dotted what looked like, yellow, breeze-blocked squash courts hastily erected within a day sometime in the early 1980s. The lean-to, sloped porch had been constructed with untreated off-cuts, which over the years had grown a thin layer of mossy green algae, making the surface akin to walking on banana-skinned black ice. The spectacular yet imposing spider web that stretched from the letterbox across the front door to a lone, naked lightbulb could have snared a flamingo in full flight and did little for my rapidly dwindling enthusiasm or mum's severe arachnophobia. Inside, the first thing that walloped us around the face was the overbearing, get-stuck-in-your-throat musty, damp smell. It was so pungent it was as if someone had inserted a mushroom into each nostril.

The hallway was also the lounge/eating area and housed two filthy once-white couches and a small, foot-by-foot TV on the wall. At the end of the utility hallway was my windowless room where two 5-foot, narrow twin beds were separated by a wood-wormed bedside table where, next to the Paw Patrol lamp, lay a well-thumbed King James V bible. The Egyptian cotton bedsheets described so decadently had been replaced with waterproof bedsheets and stained, thin, lumpy pillows. To finish off my 'deluxe family suite' was the discovery of a condom wrapper under one of the beds.

Mum's room, in comparison, was positively palatial. Her bed was at the top of the impossibly narrow staircase overlooking the communal bin area. On tip-toes, it was just possible to make out a puddle in a pothole which we agreed must be the waterside view and remaining consistent throughout, another crudely fitting waterproof double-bedsheet that covered a plastic-coated mattress. Her en-suite consisted of a shower cubicle with a sink in the corner, preventing anybody, regardless of shape, size or athleticism from being able to thoroughly shower unless they had one foot on the shower mat outside the cubicle, turning the en-suite into more of a wet room. The broken toilet seat encouraged the user to hover just above rather than risk anything delicate being caught by conventional usage. The cistern permanently and noisily refilled.

The worst road in Europe wasn't any easier to negotiate by car headlight. If anything, the shadows only highlighted precisely why the Volvo Estate lay abandoned by the wayside and why the three hundred metres to the main road took nearly fifteen minutes to complete.

When we came to a blissful halt at the end, the sight of pub lights just down the road was most welcome. The bursting car park indicated 'The Sloop's' popularity amongst the locals, and once inside, it became clear why. Rammed to the rafters were families with plates piled so high they defied gravity. The everyday, all-day, all-you-can-eat carvery buffet for £8.99 had been taken to the absolute extreme. The creativity and ingenuity of some of the builds on display demonstrated the amateur architects wasted understanding of complex structural engineering. Cauliflower cheese foundations propped up sausages which were being used as load-bearing pillars for floors of sliced chicken and beef. Giant Yorkshire puddings on top held in neatly constructed tiers of roast potatoes. Small children could have drowned in the gravy moat surrounding most masterpieces.

Aside from the carvery, the menu offered enough for us to order a drink and look for a table. Without hope of finding a vacant one inside, we made do with one out on the terrace next to a family of four eagerly waiting for the buffet queue to shorten. Such was their anticipation they had already neatly laid their cutlery on the table in front of them. Of course, one of the hazards of al fresco dining by the sea is the constant aerial threat of circling seagulls, and as mum and I mulled over the menu, we were distracted by the sudden commotion next to us. Out of the night sky, a seagull had deposited directly and squarely onto the father's fork, followed by hysteria from the children and pirate parlance from the fuming father. He cleaned his fork with his paper serviette and then put his arm in the air to attract the waitress's attention. Bizarrely, instead of asking for a replacement fork, he asked for another paper serviette as he fiddled with his soiled fork between his thumb and forefinger.

Our takeaway pizzas arrived at the same time as the daughter returned from the buffet, slightly buckled under the weight of food she had balanced precariously on her plate. Tired and hungry, we made a third trip in 2 hours along the car killing road from hell. By the time the key was pulled from the ignition for the final time that day, we both felt we'd done a shift on a heavy-duty pneumatic drill. We ended the day perched on the edge of the sofas, watching the tiny T.V., scrapping demolished pizza off the cardboard, already dreading the morning car journey.

Having found it more comfortable to sleep on the floor between the beds than forcing myself into a stress position on one of the pygmy mattresses, I woke feeling like I'd been used as a rugby tackle bag. Mum fared worse. Her warped posture had aged her by a decade and she had developed a dry, ticklish cough overnight. The wind had also changed direction and now blew in gusts of bin air, giving our villa a rotting compost, gag-inducing aroma.

After brief discussion, we agreed that we must be staying in the arsehole of the island and so with boundless determination, we reinforced the car seats with borrowed cushions and set-off on our adventure discovering hidden beaches and sleepy coastal pubs. Before we had left Wormley, mum, in an unconscious moment of clairvoyance had booked us both a Thai massage later that afternoon on the far side of the island, and so with gay abandonment, decided to head in that general direction, walking Anton en-route.

It soon became evident that the island's arsehole was more extensive than we had previously thought and seemingly inhabited almost exclusively by aging pensioners, many of whom could be found standing by the side of remote lanes, waiting for buses. The dog-friendly beach was anything but friendly. Boulders the size the world's strongest men compete to lift, lay strewn from the £1.80 per hour car park right up to the water's edge 50 metres away. A coffee kiosk at the end of the car park run by two kids of G.C.S.E. age did a roaring trade selling to a monosyllabic, hung-over wedding party whilst their disappointed children with brand new buckets and spades fought back wobbly lips and leaky eyes.

We brunched in Lidl's car park out of necessity rather than choice and continued on our magical mystery tour as leaden clouds rolled across the sky, still optimistic our sandy haven was just around the next corner. 2 hours later and we had exhausted both our buttocks and any hope of finding our island idyll that day and so punched the postcode of our Thai massage into the sat-nav.

When the sat-nav lady proudly announced we had arrived at our final destination, we had to double-check the coordinates entered, thinking there must have been an input error. Regardless of how often we revised the postcode or address, the result remained the same. With the windscreen wipers working at full capacity, we stared at the wheel-less frame of a child's long abandoned bicycle, locked to a broken drainpipe on the wall of a partially graffitied, pebble-dashed terraced house, dispiriting mum, and leaving me wondering whether the establishment was above board and legal. Standing sentry on either side of the entrance to a side alley were two four-foot plastic palm trees adorned in fairy lights. After one last google-map check on mum's phone again confirmed we were where we should be, we gingerly left the safety of the car, relying on Anton as security on the back seat, and made our way through the tropical gateway.

We were greeted by two immaculately uniformed Thai ladies, who, after asking us to remove our shoes, led us into a converted garage. Something must have been lost in translation when mum had booked us in over the phone as before us stood two beds pushed together, and on them, scattered red rose petals and two chocolate love hearts. Dozens of candles dotted around the sides gave the room a soft glow whilst Enya's greatest hits played in the background. Although I'm close to my mother, in no way, shape or form could our relationship ever be defined as romantic or sexual. Once the confusion had been clarified, we were escorted back out of the garage to stand in the rain while they busily made the appropriate adjustments inside.

On the earlier questionnaire we had been asked to complete, mum had requested a 'medium' massage and I had opted for a 'hard' one, casually confident I could take whatever pressure my 5'1", seven-stone masseuse could exert. Thirty minutes in and with my eyes bulging at the floor, I could have sworn the petite woman walking up and down my back barefoot also had a large sack of potatoes on her shoulders. As mum had generously booked us both a double massage, I had an hour and a half of being used as a human treadmill to look forward to.

When she eventually climbed off me, the painful wheezing in my chest made me think she'd fractured a rib and I'd just been the paying victim of a common physical assault. The traditional 'happy-ending' often associated with Thai massages couldn't have been further from my mind as I stared at my bloodshot eyes in the scarred mirror by the door, holding my tender sides. Mum, meanwhile, looked as though she had been dragged through a garden centre backwards and had similar difficulties dressing herself.

We both required assistance shoeing our feet and, having whispered our insincere thanks and goodbyes, supported each other back to the car, where we sat in punch-drunk silence, gazing through the wet windscreen at the dismembered bike. As we tried to come to terms with the relaxing ordeal we'd just endured, we questioned which had been worse for our bodies, the road to and from hell or paying to be pummelled by a barefoot stranger in a garage for an hour and a half.

Once the stars had subsided and I was safe to drive again, we set course for Ryde and somewhere to eat. Despite being able to drive across the entire island in an hour, diversions, road works, traffic jams, and pensioners standing perilously close by roadsides lengthened the relatively straightforward journey considerably and shortened patience equally.

Ryde was heaving, as if the whole island had decided to descend on the town that night. On the outskirts of the town itself, I was faced with one too many pointless, forgotten road closure signs, so I took the confident advice of the sat-nav lady and continued on down a quiet, one-way residential street to our targeted Indian restaurant just around the corner on the main high street. Not far down, I noticed the flashing amber lights of a highway's vehicle in the rear-view mirror which had stopped at the entrance of the street we had turned down. The first pang of doubt that rippled through my beaten body came as I watched two chaps get out and place traffic cones across the road. The second was when our car was engulfed in pedestrians of all ages whilst trying to turn left down the main street. When we pushed out onto the main road, trying to escape the hoards on the pavement, it became abundantly apparent why all the roads had been closed and what thousands of people were doing streaming around our car on a Saturday night.

My poor decision-making and rebellious reluctance to adhere to the basics of the highway code had landed us between a 'Ryde Ballet School' carnival float in front and the 'Isle of Wight – LGBT' community hoola-hooping troupe behind. On both sides of the route, 2 or 3 deep, stood families with prams and couples holding hands, smiling and waving to the slow-moving festive column. Unable to turn around or reverse, we had little choice but to reciprocate the hand-waving from behind the darkened windows of our very ordinary, slightly dirty burgundy A1 Audi as mum handed me my arse through gritted teeth. There followed one of the longest 15 minutes I've ever sat in a car, second only to the time waiting to see my mistaken superfan at the local tip. I'll never forget the expression on one enthusiastic young boy's face when he saw us; it was as if an unseen puppeteer had entered him uninvited.

We drove straight past our intended Indian, disregarding the many accusations made by the cocky sat-nav that we'd overshot our target, and so, with wrist-waving fatigue, took the earliest opportunity to escape down a side-road and head back out of town to the same Lidl's car park for the second meal of the day.

As we sat on the grubby couch in our 'villa', a quick Google search revealed we had inadvertently taken part in Ryde Carnival, the oldest carnival in the UK, dating from 1887. In one way or another, it had been an exhausting day, so much so I wasn't fazed when faced with the child's mattress in my damp cave. It turns out it was the perfect size for my body as it curled up in foetal Pompeii shock.

The following morning, try as I might, I could not straighten my back, so spent the first hour scuttling about like Gollum, gasping loudly and swearing whenever movement was required. Mum was bent double so badly her fingers were almost in constant contact with her toes, and her dry, ticklish cough had progressed into loud, whooping fits so fierce I feared she'd throw up a lung. Neither of us could feel our well-worn buttocks.

Concerned mum was displaying symptoms of full-blown pneumonia and the ongoing long-term damage inflicted by the natives and the third-world roads; we mutually conceded that for health reasons alone, we should cut our island getaway short by four days and retreat home on the next available ferry.

After one last bone-shuddering journey, we saluted the buckled blue Volvo estate a fond farewell and waited at the end of the road for an eternity as a senile, elderly gentleman, took pleasure in delaying all traffic by repeatedly bashing the button on the pedestrian key-pad he had just crossed the road to arrive at. Amid the car horns and fruity verbal instructions on where the old man should go, we slipped the lights and escaped the rising tension of the bemused motorists, thanking the powers that be when we arrived unscathed and intact at the ferry terminal.

Unlike the previous crossing, the ferry was relatively empty and the going smooth. Standing alone on the stern deck, mum, Anton, and I watched Ryde port shrink with an ever-growing sense of ease. We disembarked at Portsmouth harbour and began following the infrequent road signs back to the A3, having lost all trust in the sat-nav the night before for making us the worst float in carnival history. We must have been down nearly every road in Portsmouth trying to find the A3, only to be eventually spat out onto the busy M27. With bruised, battered buttocks and patience in low supply, the sense of relief had become a sense of accomplishment when we pulled into the drive at home. In four days, I have never sat in a car for longer and done so few miles than on that holiday. It was good to be home.

It was good to be home…for 6 seconds anyway. Before I'd had a chance to release the seat-belt, mum realised she was without her handbag and must have left it on deck when we were saying grateful goodbyes to the Isle of shite. The panicked phone call to the ferry company was made in full expectation of receiving disappointing news, but astonishingly not only did it go well, it was a complete success. The more than charming customer service operator contacted the boat skipper, who then found the handbag and secured it in their safe, ready for mum to collect when it docked back at Portsmouth. So, we were back on the road again without even having the luxury of pulling the key from the ignition.

True to their word, mum's handbag and its contents were fully intact and waiting for us to collect at the terminal, earning the employee who handed mum her bag much deserved praise and earnest gratitude for a faultless service.

Having carefully adhered to the road signs earlier, only to end up travelling along a motorway in the opposite direction, we agreed to give the sat-nav another opportunity to redeem itself, seeing as it couldn't do any worse than the national signage. And once again, an hour later, we were proved wrong. Not only did we find ourselves joining the same motorway, but after another endless diversion, we were somehow 20 miles closer to Southampton and 20 miles further from home. It was as if the northbound M27 had an inescapable, magnetic tractor beam reeling us in.

We managed to narrowly avoid the clutches of Southampton's outer suburbs at rush hour by taking the third alternative, longer scenic route offered by the disgraced sat-nav, preferring any view to that of more stationary brake lights. When we finally arrived at our front door, we moved like stiff extras from Michael Jackson's 'Thriller' video. From what should have been a door-to-door jaunt of just over two hours took just under seven and completed what had essentially been a 3-day driving holiday. We hadn't wasted our time away though. We'd been an unofficial float in the UK's oldest carnival, had super-humanly strong Thai women use us for their daily workout, had mum nearly succumb to severe respiratory complications and left both of us with a reluctance to sit down.

ANALYSE THIS

'When a woman has not had sex for a long time, she turns'
– Freud

As MUCH AS I loved exploring our green and pleasant land, I was looking forward to the next chapter of my life and getting my teeth stuck into the experiential counselling course. The college I was attending had also seen my cousin and mother pass through its esteemed corridors years earlier, making it almost a family tradition. When enrolment day arrived, I made the 20-minute drive feeling like it was my first day at school all over again. As I wandered around searching for the elusive classroom, I could imagine mum doing the same in the swinging sixties and last probable decade the walls were painted.

I finally found the classroom, or rather people standing outside it. Having confirmed I was in the right place, I asked a 60-something-year-old fellow student why everyone was in the corridor and not in the classroom, and just like school, I was told we weren't allowed entry until the tutor invited us in. Right on the minute, the door opened, and the same aromatic woman who had interviewed me held it open as we filed past her in silence.

We each took a seat in a semi-circle that faced two chairs at the front in a neglected, jaded room. An array of seashells dangled on strings from the peeling ceiling above and covering the walls, almost child-like paper montages of different mental-health disorders. Sitting at a desk in front of a laptop with her broad bison's back to us, our second tutor, who, when introduced, raised the back of her hand in acknowledgement and continued with whatever she was doing on the computer. When it was our turn to introduce ourselves, we had to do it through the medium of song and dance. One by one, blushing faces took to their feet and twirled uncomfortably whilst singing their name. It was chastening to perform and even more torturous to watch. There was a momentary concern for the eldest in our group when she thought she'd slipped a disk whilst enthusiastically pirouetting, requiring assistance back to her seat and a glass of water.

The next topic were the rules and regulations and what was expected of the students. Firstly, to prevent cliques from forming, social interaction between students was strictly forbidden. No telephone calls, no emails, no messages, no nothing. In class, personal information should exclusively be shared in the break-out groups and not in general group discussion. Any breach would automatically result in an immediate warning and a 2nd offence, expulsion from the course. Next, no student may remain in the room at break times and must wait outside the room until called. Tardiness of attendance and homework would be punished with an official warning. Two warnings and you're out. The tutors would closely monitor the 100 compulsory sessions of external personal therapy and if they thought progression wasn't swift enough, which I never understood, considering it's a confidential conversation between client and therapist, they have the authority to discount any sessions undertaken when the student has to restart with another counsellor. (Each counselling session ranges between £50-£90). We were sternly told that hot drinks during class were categorically not permitted as the two tutors regularly recharged their coffee mugs from the kettle at the front. Lastly, whether the student completes the course is entirely at their discretion. If, for whatever reason deemed unworthy, the student would have to apply the following year and undergo the same selection process; no refunds would be offered. It had already cost each of us £2750 to have the privilege of being belittled by one woman who smelt like she was having an affair with a horse and the other who hadn't yet had the decency to face the class and was eating her seat. In all my years, even when I was at school or at home with my stepfather, Barrie the bastard, have I ever witnessed such a grotesque display of power and control. They were queens of their crumbling kingdom, and we were their lowly, dependent subjects who knew nothing, and they made sure we knew it.

Of the sixteen in class, three were men, accurately reflecting the industry's gender ratio, whilst the average age must have been around 60, with me being the youngest. We were divided into four groups of four based on personality types from our little introductory jig, which smacked of judgement on a course and career which actively discourages judgements. Each group was allocated a small side room where we were sent for skills practice under the supervision of the tutors, who popped in and out intermittently. My group consisted of the two eldest ladies and one of the other tattooed chaps who was already on a warning for letting it slip in class that he was a builder, breaking the rule of divulging personal details in general class. As punishment, he also had the unenviable task of being a counsellor in the first roleplay. Before he'd even opened his mouth, he was reprimanded a second time for not removing three small random, clay skulls on the floor in the corner and then a third time, for not straightening a curtain. The final insult came when he tried to introduce himself, only to be shut down for not being confident in his delivery. She left the room shaking her head, and the poor builder on the verge of tears. She returned to tell the builder his homework was to write a reflective 1,500-word document on what he'd learned in his skills practice.

Because we weren't allowed to communicate on a communication course, lunch was a strange, solemn affair. Whilst most of us sat in the canteen, smiling at each other in awkward silence, the builder could be seen outside chain-smoking and arguing with himself. Sure enough, when we returned to class, we were given a strong 'OUT!' with a dismissive hand wave and had to wait in the corridor until the door was opened to us. The afternoon was conducted in silence as paperwork was distributed and explained. If any questions arose, students were to raise their arm. Some had to change arms while they waited patiently for their name to be called.

Being back in the classroom hadn't been as joyful as I had envisaged and made me appreciate the independence that Zoom gatherings offer. Also, after witnessing the builder getting savagely torn to shreds, I worried how I would manage under the same circumstances, whether I was mentally robust enough to take such a personal stripping down.

TWO DAYS LATER, I attended a head and neck cancer survivor seminar hosted by the Royal Surrey. Much of the day was difficult to listen to, especially when the maxillofacial surgeon outlined the long-term side-effects of my particular treatment. Regardless whether I persevered with the painful mouth-stretches twice a day for the rest of my life, there was the very real possibility that one day, without warning, my jaw would permanently clamp shut, never to reopen, thus forever preventing speech and requiring all sustenance thereafter to pass down a tube directly into my stomach. None of the speakers expressed any optimism and I left feeling as though I had a time-bomb in my mouth. From that day forth, each and every morning, the first thing I do, even before opening my eyes, is see whether I've become mute overnight. The whole day had rocked my recovering mind and sent shock-waves of self-doubt rippling through me.

THE 2ND WEEK at college confirmed that I couldn't continue the course. After being invited in, the tutors at the front openly and loudly discussed a private client one of the tutors had seen the previous night. Not only did they entirely disregard the confidentiality agreement, but they also went straight to his sexual attraction, which made the larger lady chuckle childishly behind her hand. When the tutor/counsellor told her there was definitely a sexual connection between the two of them that would need to be explored at 'length', the other giddy tutor nearly pissed her marquee pants. It was grim.

What hadn't been previously discussed or broached was the tremendous cost of qualifying to be a BACP registered counsellor. Over the next 18 months, the course, learning materials, personal therapy, supervision sessions, and agency placements would likely be in excess of £10,000. Considering it's an unregulated industry, that was a lot of money to get on a register, and money I simply didn't have. Looking around at my ashen-faced peers, I clearly wasn't the only one dumbfounded. The day concluded with the drooling horsey tutor asking us to please bring in a tea towel to cover our laps and some wet wipes as we were studying Freud the following week. The heavier tutor, who had repositioned herself back in front of the computer, sniggered so vigorously I thought her creaking chair would be swallowed at any moment.

I just didn't have the mental fortitude to be denigrated by two immature, sex-obsessed, self-righteous queens and pay exorbitant amounts to have my balls in their eager hands for the next two years. So here I am, sitting on the edge of my bed at another crossroads, with Anton lazing beside me, staring out of my bedroom window and occasionally talking to my leafy friends, Christina, Carina, and Celina. In the far distance, I can see a red, hot air balloon gently ascending heavenward, and in the foreground, a robin is slowly but surely inching its way across the roof of the shed toward my hopeful, extended forefinger. This afternoon I have to stop by the tip on the way to a booked massage in Godalming before doing some food shopping and finishing with a quick pint. Tomorrow morning, I have a dog walk, a six-month surveillance scan in a hospital gown and in the afternoon, I'm travelling down to Devon for an overnight stay in a remote village. Mum's downstairs googling holidays.

What could possibly go wrong?

EPILOGUE

When I first sat down to write this, my initial objective was simple and straightforward; ego, immortality. Without a partner, descendants, or legacy, I had real difficulty getting to grips with the idea that the only evidence that I lived would be a quickly forgotten and overgrown headstone. In the months it's taken me to write this instalment, that objective has been revisited and revised several times.

Notwithstanding *Lady Luck and Me*'s modest success, much of what I wrote was a grievous error in judgment, losing me far more friends and good people than I gained. To those I recklessly and needlessly wronged, I offer my long overdue deepest apologies. Arrogance and ignorance are not adequate defences.

From my diagnosis on 16/12/19 to walking out of that tiny windowless room of which the ceiling I knew so well on 10/02/22, I had had over 125 cancer-related appointments, an incalculable mileage, and countless hours of conversations with dozens of doctors. At the time of writing, there have been less than 30 recorded cases of my particular sarcoma, the last one being in Bangladesh in the early 1970's. They have now established it had, in all likelihood, been growing since birth.

Cancer has been the most positively transformative episode of my life, a cliché which you've probably read a thousand times. I give far fewer 'fucks' now than I did before, which has led to the highs not being quite so high and the lows, thankfully not so low. It's brought an element of peace and stability through an inner strength, and has left me safe in the knowledge that very few things in life will be as stressful, apart from going to the local tip or having a massage. There weren't any eureka moments or epiphanies but rather gradual changes over the months and although it went largely under the radar at the time, I feel the changes have been profound, so much so that I view my life in two distinct halves, pre-cancer and post-cancer. It has shone a light and exposed parts of me, good and bad, which I don't think would have been revealed in any other experience. For that alone, I'm grateful to the disease.

Despite occasionally frightening myself in the mirror and witnessing strangers diving into bushes to avoid me, I'm not as self-conscious as I used to be before my life changing facial injuries. I've decided against reconstruction or cosmetic surgery partly because of the hospital gowns but mainly because this is who I am now. That's not to say I'll be eating out anytime soon; that remains a meal too far.

Cancer and depression do share one very unsavoury, distinct characteristic; loneliness. Both effect and drive a wedge between you, life, and your loved ones. Of the two diseases, in my own unique experience, depression at its worst has been far more painful than at any stage of my cancer diagnosis and subsequent treatment. It sounds absurd to say, but personally and for context, I'd bite your hand off to have the worst of my cancer over the worst of any depressive episode. I actually think my experiences as a depressive greatly helped in preparing me for the psychological side of cancer. Many of the feelings of anxiety and fears for the future, although more concentrated, were nothing new. I never imagined that one day, I'd be thanking depression for making my life easier.

Have I found purpose? Have I found peace? I find purpose in pursuing peace is the answer. I now know peace is possible, albeit through the worst personal news and maybe as a result of shock, but the sensation, however fleeting, was real enough to inspire that that state of blissful contentment is somewhere within me. If I've felt it once, I can again and hope the next time will be under happier, healthier conditions.

As for the future, who knows what Lady Luck has in store. Airport security will be a problem, as will French kissing and dentists but as long as I have the power of speech and means of communication, I still very much wish to use it for counselling purposes. Eating will forever be a trial. Having said that, I'm grateful for each and every meal that I'm still able to cram in my mouth, liquified food delivered through a plastic tube into my stomach won't have the same appeal.

Finally, and most importantly, my thanks. There were many times when I almost abandoned writing this altogether. Crippling thoughts of self-indulgence and self-doubt consumed many fruitless hours. The one constant motivation that kept me writing was people or, to be more precise, those people who directly and indirectly kept me alive, and so by the end, my focus had shifted from wanting the world to know I existed to wanting the world to know how very grateful I am to those people. This book was finished for them and is intended to be a permanent record and reminder of my eternal gratitude.

My mother – for your unwavering support and unconditional love. For your understanding, patience, wisdom and compassion. I learn from you each and every day and know that having you as my mother has been my very best of luck. I love you.

Emma Kendall – for the fondest, life-lasting memories and always being there no matter how many times I disappoint.

Charmian D'Aubosson – for always being there and making me a very proud little brother. I love you mate.

Anton – for getting me out, being the finest companion and very best of friends.

Clair Blackaby – for keeping my head above water when I was ready to sink below, many times.

Debbie Holmes – for the very finest of introductions.

Billie-Joe Duddell – for never letting me down when called upon.

Sandie Titheridge– for the size of your heart. The world needs more people like you.

Sarah Davies – for always making me feel one of the family.

Pea – for your friendship, laughter and love which I never deserved.

Isabella and Finlay – for giving me a genuine sense of joy.

Harriet Weston – for your friendship, belief and teaching me the power of words, and their misuse.

J-C Nunes – for giving the best hugs.

Witley CC – for giving suitable reason to be sunburnt, angry and in God's garden with the most excellent people.

MacMillan – for life-saving intervention and counselling. Heroes.

Royal Surrey County Hospital – for treating the patient with dignity and saving my life twice.

The Royal Marsden – for treating the cancer.

Printed in Great Britain
by Amazon

21595766R00123